Frontiers in Vestibular and Oculo-Motor Research

Liber-Amicorum in Honour of Prof. Hans Engström

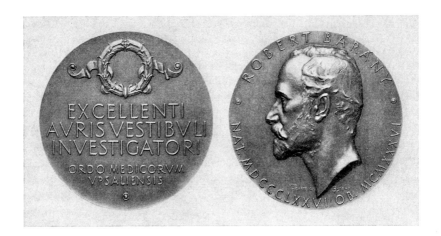

Volume Editor
J. Stahle, Uppsala

71 figures and 19 tables, 1979

S. Karger · Basel · München · Paris · London · New York · Sydney

Advances in Oto-Rhino-Laryngology

Vol. 23: Pediatric Otorhinolaryngology. Ed.: B. Jazbi, Kansas City, Mo.
VIII + 206 p., 101 fig., 1 cpl., 16 tab., 1978. ISBN 3–8055–2674–1
Vol. 24: Modern Methods of Radiology in ORL. Selected papers of the VIIth
International Congress of Radiology in ORL, Copenhagen 1976.
Eds.: S. Brünner, Copenhagen and P.E. Andersen, Odense.
VIII + 196 p., 145 fig., 15 tab., 1978. ISBN 3–8055–2707–1

National Library of Medicine Cataloging in Publication
Bárány Society
Frontiers in vestibular and oculo-motor research :
liber-amicorum in honour of Professor Hans Engström /
volume editor, J. Stahle. – – Basel ; New York : Karger, 1979.
(Advances in oto-rhino-laryngology ; v. 25)
Proceedings of the Bárány Society ordinary meeting in Uppsala, June 1–3, 1978.
1. Labyrinth Diseases – congresses   2. Oculomotor Muscles – congresses
3. Oculomotor Nerve – congresses   4. Vestibular Apparatus – congresses
I. Stahle, Jan, ed.   II. Engström, Hans   III. Title   IV. Series
WV 255 B225f 1978
ISBN 3–8055–2988–0

Frontiers in Vestibular and Oculo-Motor Research

Advances in Oto-Rhino-Laryngology

Vol. 25

Series Editor
C. R. Pfaltz, Basel

S. Karger · Basel · München · Paris · London · New York · Sydney

Contents

Contents

Contents   VII

There have been few scientists in our field whose research work has been so versatile and at the same time so profound. *Hans Engström's* research spans over a very large field, with morphology predominating. His first major work, which was also his doctoral thesis, was published in 1940 and was entitled 'Über das Vorkommen der Otosklerose nebst experimentellen Studien über chirurgische Behandlung der Krankheit'. At the beginning of the 1950s his interest became focused on the ultrastructure of the internal ear, which led to a number of important observations. The surface specimen technique was another innovation which has gained wide application, especially in studies of cell changes caused by noise and ototoxic antibiotics. During the 1970s his research has been concentrated on the deleterious effects of noise on the internal ear, as documented by scanning electron micrographs of extremely high quality.

Hans Engström's research laboratories have become an important school for advanced studies of the internal ear, and have given inspiration to many collaborators and students, who have carried this line of research further. These include, among many others, Ades, Angelborg, Axelsson, Ballantyne, Bergström, Bredberg, Hawkins, Kellerhals, Lindeman, Rosenhall, Spoendlin, Watanuki and Wersäll.

Hans Engström's creative research has received considerable international praise, as witnessed by the numerous medals and prizes which he has received, including the Purkinje medal (1964), the Shambaugh prize (1967), the Guyot prize (1969), the Paris city bronze medal (1974), the medal of the Uppsala Medical Association and the Gunnar Holmgren medal. To these we may also add the honorary membership of the Royal Society of Medicine, Otolaryngology, and membership of several other international societies.

It is the sincere hope of the members of the Bárány Society and of *Hans Engström's* previous and present colleagues that he will be able to continue his purposeful, fundamental and imaginative research for many years to come.

Jan Stahle
President of the Bárány Society

Adv. Oto-Rhino-Laryng., vol. 25, pp. 1–6 (Karger, Basel 1979)

The Labyrinth of the American Bullfrog

H. Engström, B. Engström and K. Watanuki

Department of Otolaryngology, University Hospital, Uppsala

Introduction

The American bullfrog *(Rana catesbiana)* has been subject to several investigations during the years. Recently the interest has considerably increased [1, 3], because such frogs will be used for studies on labyrinth function in weightlessness.

In cooperation with *T. Gualthierotti* in Pittsburgh we have started a careful analysis, in a series of adult bullfrogs, of the vestibular sensory regions. This study primarily aims at a population study of all the sensory regions in the frog labyrinth. The study has been made using light and electron microscopy.

Methods

The light microscopic study has been made using a technique developed by *K. Watanuki* who has made this count of cells in specimens prepared with his silver nitrate method. This method permits a distinction of the cell borders of individual cells and the whole surface of each sensory region can be studied in micrographs. By comparing microphotographs and specimens as they are seen under the microscope we believed that we could get reliable results concerning the cell populations. As will be discussed below care must be taken to use other techniques also to get reliable results. For our population studies we also used scanning electron microscopy (SEM) applying methods, described in several of our earlier publications [2]. By careful preparation it is possible to get specimens from each individual sensory area in which every single cell can be observed and counted. By this technique we are now comparing the light and SEM specimens. It seems clear that the SEM study gives truer results and the differences from the light microscopic results may amount to 30%. For a reliable population study we therefore believe that SEM is to be preferred.

Our cell counts were made simultaneously with a transmission electron microscopic study of the sensory epithelium and of nerve branches. The exact methodology which has followed ordinary techniques used in SEM and TEM will be described in a more extensive publication.

Results

Light microscopic Study. All sensory regions (fig. 1) have been photo-graphed and a complete cell count made. According to these counts, Lagena contains about 6,200 cells.

	Light microscopy	SEM
Lagena	6,200	
Macula utriculi	9,350	
Macula sacculi	4,000	3,600
Crista lateralis	3,430	
Crista anterior	4,320	
Crista posterior	4,400	
Crista neglecta	2,470	1,400, 1,700

It can be of interest to compare these figures with a parallel study on macula utriculi in guinea pig where macula utriculi contains about 9,200 cells.

SEM Study. It is possible to prepare the sensory regions so that their whole surface or parts of it can be extremely well visualized by SEM. A whole macula can often be beautifully prepared and individual cells or cell groups studied in detail. In the study of the crista certain problems arise. It is often difficult to get a quality comparable to the one we get in the maculae and this partly depends upon the presence of much longer stereo- and kinocilia on the crista. We are working on this problem and it is possible that population studies will have to rely upon experiments where the cilia have been separated from the cell surface. In figure 2A there is given an example of how SEM can demonstrate the appearance of the surface of a small group of cells and their surface organelles. This micro-graph is only a small portion of a whole macula utriculi where the quality is comparable over the whole surface.

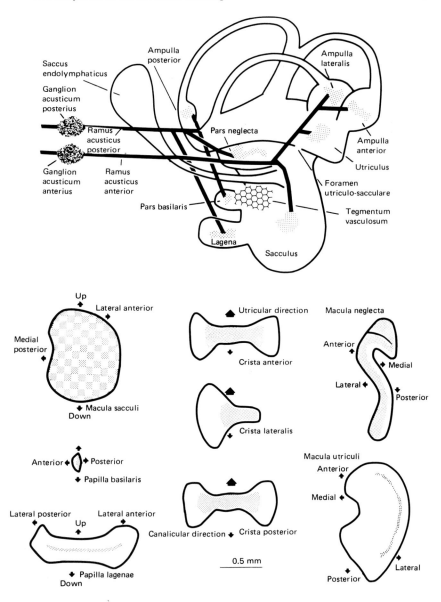

Fig. 1. General arrangement of sensory regions and their nerve fibers in the American bullfrog, *Rana catesbiana.*

The SEM study, which will be extensive, is continued, but has already demonstrated that it is possible to get very reliable quantitative results concerning cell population studies. It has also given important information concerning form, size and arrangement of kino- and stereocilia and of other surface organelles.

Transmission Electron Microscopic (TEM) Study. We have had certain problems in acquiring very high quality TEM material in these frogs. It is common to get a certain shrinkage in some specimens and this constitutes a problem which has to be overcome by improved technique. In an evaluation of small structural changes it is necessary to work with a very reliable preparation technique. That this is possible is evident from the good results seen in several of our specimens.

The basic structure of the vestibular sensory cells shows a good resemblance to sensory cells of type II (according to Wersäll). All the sensory cells are provided with one kinocilium and several stereocilia. The length and form of both kino- and stereocilia may vary, not only between different sensory regions, but also between individual cells in one sensory area. This variation depends on a specific pattern similar from one animal to the next.

The sensory cells are richly provided with nerve endings mainly at their lower portion but synaptic contacts are also seen high up above the nuclear region. The sensory cells contain numerous large, round electron-dense, bodies surrounded by transmitter granules. They appear mainly close to a region of synaptic contact, but they may also be found in the cell cytoplasm without any contact with the cell surface. Thus they may even be found close to the nucleus.

It is also common to see that one nerve ending can form contact with more than one sensory cell (fig. 2B) and that clusters of synaptic bodies may be found close to the nerve ending in more than one cell.

The sensory epithelium is richly provided with nerve fibers and nerve endings. The largest number is of the nongranulated type. In all areas we have observed granulated endings also and these granulated, presumably efferent, endings are very large and numerous in certain regions. These are

---

Fig. 2. A SEM micrograph of the epithelial surface in Macula utriculi. Large arrow indicates a kinocilium, one on each cell. Small arrow points at stereocilia, which here are rather short. *B* Nerve ending (Ne) in contact with two sensory cells. The arrows indicate synaptic bodies and synaptic areas in the upper cell. *A* = × 6,500; *B* = × 24,000.

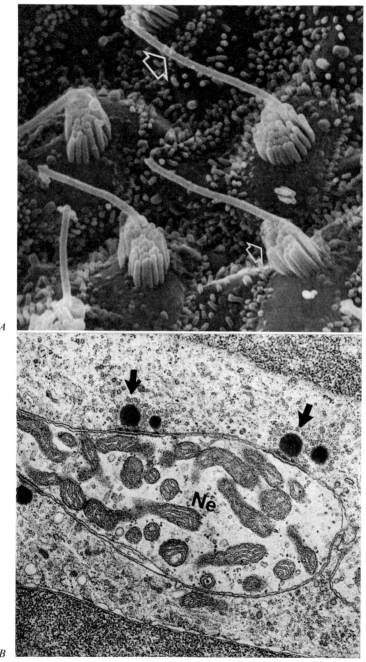

A

B

now being further examined using different nerve-staining methods for light and electron microscopy.

Summary

The labyrinth of the American bullfrog *(Rana catesbiana)* has been studied by aid of light and electron microscopy. Cell counts and sensory area mapping has been made and it has been shown that scanning electron microscopy is the most appropriate technique at present for cell counts.

References

1   Cohen, G.M.; Reschke, M., and Ryan, P.: Saccular hair cells in the adult bullfrog *Rana catesbiana*. ARO Meet. 1978.
2   Boyde, A. and Vesely, P.: Proc. Annu. Scanning Electron Microscopy Symposia, p. 266 (1972).
3   Lewis, E.R.: Differences in the receptors of the auditory organs in the frog. ARO Meet. 1978.

Prof. H. Engström, MD, Department of Otolaryngology, University Hospital, S-750 14 Uppsala (Sweden)

Adv. Oto-Rhino-Laryng., vol. 25, pp. 7–11 (Karger, Basel 1979)

Genesis and Maturation of Vestibular Hair Cells

Matti Anniko, Hans Nordemar and Jan Wersäll

Department of Otolaryngology, Karolinska Sjukhuset and King Gustaf V
Research Institute, Karolinska Institutet, Stockholm

Introduction

The comparative embryologic development in mammals has been of
great value for the understanding of human conditions. The introduction of
in vitro techniques for inner ear studies offers a new tool in developmental
investigations [*Fell,* 1928; *Friedmann,* 1965; *Van De Water and Ruben,* 1971].

In the present study the hair cell development of the crista ampullaris
in vivo and *in vitro* was analyzed ultrastructurally. The otocyst was explanted to *in vitro* conditions at various stages of development and followed
to a maturation corresponding to partus.

Material and Methods

For the *in vitro* study, groups of otocysts from the CBA/CBA mouse were explanted on the 13th and 16th gestational day, respectively, and followed not only by direct
observation and photodocumentation but also by daily fixation of 6–8 otocysts for morphological investigation. The *in vivo* group of inner ears comprised otocysts taken for
fixation each day from the 13th gestational day until partus on the 21st gestational day.

A detailed description of the organ culture technique and morphological investigation
has been given by *Anniko et al.* [1979] and *Nordemar and Anniko* [1979].

Results

Organogenesis

The 13th day inner ear anlage is cystic but slightly elongated. During
the following 2 days the vestibular part is formed with semicircular canals

and ampullar widenings. The cochlear partition also develops, though without complete coiling. The gross development *in vitro* follows the *in vivo* conditions but is slightly delayed, approximately 12 h but sometimes up to 24 h. Histologic sections through the ampullar regions show frequent mitotic cells during the 13th, 14th and sometimes also the 15th gestational day but few are observed thereafter (fig. 1) Because of the delay in development following explantation, the *in vitro* group of otocysts showed mitosis on the 16th gestational day more often than was found in embryos in uterine life.

Explantation of the 16th gestational day inner ear anlage revealed a rather mature organ by means of gross morphology which remained comparatively unchanged *in vitro* (fig. 3). The cochlear end, however, showed increased coiling.

Cytodifferentiation

Cells differentiating into hair cells have undergone their terminal mitosis near the otocyst lumen. The cell population facing the lumen by the 14th gestational day is no longer homogenous. Cells are found with regularly arranged microvilli at their apex (fig. 2). On the 15th gestational day, or at a corresponding age if the inner ear anlage has been explanted on the 13th gestational day, sensory hairs can be identified. All cells, which reach the surface of the organ are provided with microvilli. The developing sensory hairs, however, became regularly arranged on the cell surface, thickened and increase in length.

Fig. 1. Light microscopy (LM). 13th gestational day inner ear. Section through the vestibular part of the inner ear anlage. The formation of the crista ampullaris is indicated by an asterisk (×). Frequent mitotic cells occur near the lumen (arrows).

Fig. 2. Electron microscopy (EM). Crista ampullaris. 14th gestational day inner ear anlage. Sensory hairs are identified but the hair cell lacks a cuticular plate.

Fig. 3. LM. 16th gestational day inner ear explant cultured 1 day *in vitro*. The cochlear and vestibular parts are clearly visible.

Fig. 4. EM. Crista ampullaris. 17th gestational day inner ear developed *in vivo*. The cuticular plate has developed in the hair cell. Rootlets penetrate into the cuticle.

Fig. 5. Crista ampullaris. 18th gestational day inner ear anlage. Afferent nerve endings are identified and also synaptic bodies have formed.

Fig. 6. LM. Crista ampullaris. 16th gestational day inner ear cultured 4 days *in vitro*. A layer of hair cells has developed and also the secretory/reabsorptive areas around the sensory epithelium can be identified. The supporting cells constitute 1–2 layers below the hair cell layer.

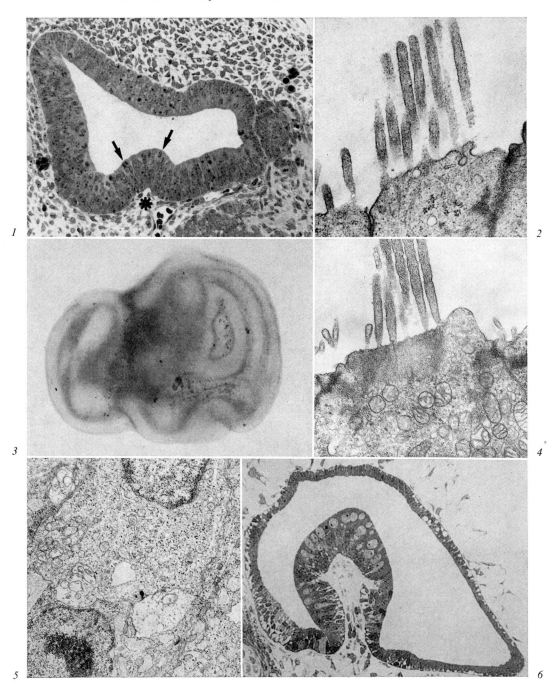

The kinocilium, initially irregularly located on the hair cell surface, is always found at the cell periphery by the 16th gestational day. The cuticular plate is formed on the 16th and 17th days *in vivo* (fig. 4). Afferent nerve terminals were identified on the 17th gestational day *in vivo* (fig. 5). On the 19th gestational day *in vivo,* hair cells were observed either with a tall columnar (rod-shape) structure and rather minimal adjacent afferent nerve terminals and hair cells with a more flask-shaped configuration having large afferent nerve endings. On the 20th gestational day efferent nerve endings were identified with certainty but nerve endings with a more vesicular content as compared with adjacent nerve terminals could be traced already on the 18th gestational day of *in vivo* development.

The 16th day inner ear explant contained already many hair cells but their number increased with culture time (fig. 6). The further development *in vitro* included formation of nerve endings and cytological transformation into a more mature configuration including nuclear migration towards the basal part of the cell – all in agreement with the *in vivo* development.

Groups of otocysts were explanted on the 13th gestational day being devoid of the adjacent stato-acoustic ganglion which had been separated from the inner ear anlage at the microdissection. Hair cells still developed and differentiated in the same way as in the *in vivo* group of inner ears. Nerve endings were, however, not identified. There was no delay in hair cell development as compared with otocysts explanted at the same age but with the adjacent ganglion intact.

Discussion

In normal fetal development, both vestibular and cochlear sensory epithelia are formed. Also in the *in vitro* environment undifferentiated epithelium develops into structures closely resembling those formed *in vivo*.

At the time of explantation of the 13th gestational day otocyst the presumptive vestibular epithelium consisted of cells that were undifferentiated, pseudostratified and rapidly proliferating. The developmental changes *in vitro* were parallel to those that occurred *in vivo* with formation of a vestibular type of hair cell. Full structural differentiation of vestibular hair cells occurred, also without the establishment of neuroepithelial contact at the synaptic level.

The 16th gestational day explant had already undergone most of its differentiation except for the ingrowth of the nervous system. Similar results were reported by *Van De Water et al.* [1977] concerning the hair cells in the macula utriculi describing progress in differentiation before any nerve fibers had reached the sensory cells. Furthermore, we found that the hair cell differentiation in organ culture of the developing crista ampullaris of the 16th gestational day inner ear anlage was almost identical with the *in vivo* development.

Summary

The embryologic development *in vivo* and *in vitro* of mammalian hair cells in the crista ampullaris was continuously followed with regard to structural differentiation and maturation from the terminal mitosis to the morphological condition at partus or equivalent age *in vitro*. Otocysts were explanted both early and late during embryologic development: 13th and 16th gestation day, respectively. Both in fetal life and during *in vitro* conditions, the surface structures of the developing hair cell with regular arrangement of kinocilium/stereocilia were first differentiated, followed by a cytologic transformation intracellularly and subsequent development of nerve endings. Hair cells were able to develop without any morphologic contact with the nervous system. The afferent nerve system developed before the efferent nerve system (CBA/CBA mouse).

References

Anniko, M.; Nordemar, H., and Van De Water, T.R.: Embryogenesis of the inner ear. I. Development and differentiation of the mammalian crista ampullaris *in vivo* and *in vitro*. Arch. Otol. Rhinol. Laryng. (in press, 1979).

Fell, H.B.: Development *in vitro* of the isolated otocyst of the embryonic fowl. Arch. exp. Zellforsch. *7:* 69–81 (1928).

Friedmann, I.: The ear; in Willmer, Cells and tissues in culture, vol. 2, pp. 521–547 (Academic Press, London 1965).

Nordemar, H. and Anniko, M.: Late embryologic development and maturation *in vitro* of the hair cells in the mammalian crista ampullaris (to be published, 1979).

Van De Water, T.R. and Ruben, R.J.: Organ culture of the mammalian inner ear. Acta oto-lar. *71:* 303–312 (1971).

Van De Water, T.R.; Anniko, M.; Nordemar, H., and Wersäll, J.: Embryonic development of the sensory cells in the macula utriculi of mouse. Colloques INSERM Symp. *68:* 25–36 (1977).

M. Anniko, MD, Karolinska Institutet, Department of Otolaryngology, Karolinska Sjukhuset and King Gustaf V Research Institute, S-104 01 Stockholm (Sweden)

Adv. Oto-Rhino-Laryng., vol. 25, pp. 12–16 (Karger, Basel 1979)

Pathological Actin in Vestibular Hair Cells of the Waltzing Guinea Pig[1]

Å. Flock, H. Cheung and J. Wersäll[2]

Department of Physiology II, Karolinska Institutet; Department of Otolaryngology, Karolinska Sjukhuset, Stockholm, and Department of Biomathematics, University of Alabama in Birmingham, Birmingham, Ala.

Introduction

Several forms of inner ear disease which lead to vestibular dysfunction or deafness involve pathological alterations in the sensory hairs which project from the apical surface of the receptor cells. Among these is a hereditary defect in the guinea pig characterized by a waltzing behavior and hearing loss [6,9]. In the vestibular system 'giant' hairs develop by fusion of stereocilia [2]. Typically, *Ernstson et al.* [2] find needle-shaped inclusion bodies in hair cells Type I [16]. These grow in an unrestricted fashion, pushing aside the nucleus and eventually penetrating the basal cell membrane contributing to cell death.

Because of their similarity to the core of stereocilia we suspected that the needles were composed by actin, as are the stereocilia [4]. This was investigated with the technique of decoration of actin filaments with myosin subfragment 1 [8].

[1] Supported by grants from the Swedish Medical Research Council (04X-02461 and 12X-00720), US National Institute of Health (AM-14589), Söderbergs Stiftelse, Bergvalls Stiftelse and Swärds Stiftelse.

[2] We are grateful to *Britta Flock* and *Yvonne Hoppe* for excellent technical assistance and to *AnnChristine Grundin* for her secretarial work.

Fig. 1. After treatment with the detergent Triton X-100 to disrupt membranes, the stereocilia and the intracellular needle-shaped inclusion body remain in place. × 23,000.

Fig. 2. Filaments inside stereocilia become labelled with myosin subfragment 1 and are thus identified as actin. × 84,000.

Fig. 3. Cytoplasmic needles are also identified as actin by labelling with S-1 fragments. × 84,000.

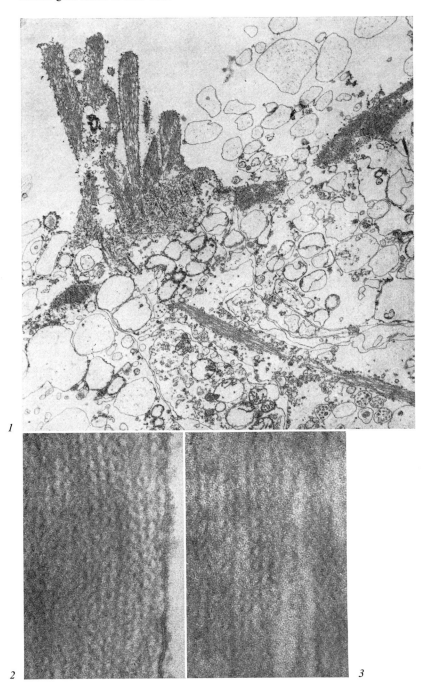

Material and Methods

Unfixed crista ampullares of waltzing guinea pigs were treated for 10 min with 0.1% Triton X-100 in Ringer's solution. This was in order to partly demembranate cells so that S-1 fragments would gain access to actin filaments. Subfragment 1 prepared from rabbit myosin [10] was used for incubation of crista as described elsewhere [4]. Fixation was done in 2% glutaraldehyde with 2 mM MgCl$_2$ buffered to pH 6.4 with cacodylate buffer. After postfixation with 1% osmic acid in the same buffer, the tissue was either mordanted with 1% tannic acid [12] or it was block impregnated with 1% uranyl acetate. Sections of Epon-embedded tissue were cut with a diamond knife on an LKB Ultrotome, stained with lead citrate and uranyl acetate and examined in a Zeiss EM 9 or a Philips 400 electron microscope.

Results

Treatment with Triton X-100 disrupts cell membranes but leaves cellular organelles reasonably in place and identifiable. Figure 1 shows a Type I hair cell with apical stereocilia and a needle-shaped inclusion body in the apical cytoplasm.

Filaments within the giant hairs become labelled after incubation with S-1 fragments, showing the serrated appearance typical of decorated actin (fig. 2). Arrowheads point down towards the cell body.

Filaments are evident also within the needles, they too are decorated by S-1 fragments, but arrowheads here point up towards the cuticular plate and away from the main cell body (fig. 3).

Discussion

Actin and myosin are the main contractile proteins in muscle cells, sliding along each other to produce shortening of the muscle. During recent years actin has been demonstrated in several nonmuscle cells, usually taking part in motile functions but also serving as mechanical support structures [5]. In nonmuscle cells, reaction of the actin is not necessarily with myosin but may be with other proteins [1] or may involve changes of actin itself from one structural form to another [14]. In certain cells, actin forms part of labile dynamic systems where polymerization of actin monomers into filaments take place as a physiological response [7, 11, 13, 15].

The appearance of abberant actin filaments in the cytoplasm of hair cells in waltzing guinea pigs indicates a loss of control of genetically determined actin polymerization. In their relation to the cuticular plate the need-les are like upside-down stereocilia, their actin filaments having opposite polarities. It is interesting to note that this makes the system similar to the sarcomere of skeletal muscle fibers having two sets of actin filaments point-ing towards a central A-band.

The apparent stiffness of the cytoplasmic needle, expressed by com-pression of the nucleas and extrusion of the basal cell membrane [2] agrees well with the observation that unfixed stereocilia are quite stiff structures [3]. Therefore, actin filaments in the needles may be packed in a manner similar to that in stereocilia.

Summary

Vestibular type I hair cells in the waltzing guinea pig contain needle-shaped inclusion bodies which grow in an uncontrolled fashion associated with the destruction of the cell. The needles are shown to be composed by filaments of actin, a protein identified in the electron microscope by its ability to bind subfragment 1 of myosin. Whereas actin filaments in stereocilia are oriented down towards the cell body, filaments in the needles point up towards the cuticular plate. The hereditary lesion appears to be associated with a defective control of polymerization of actin into filaments.

References

1   De Rosier, D.; Mandelkow, E.; Sillman, A.; Tilney, L., and Kane, R.: Structure of actin-containing filaments from two types of nonmuscle cells. J. molec. Biol. *113:* 679–695 (1977).

2   Ernstsson, S.; Lundquist, P.-G.; Wedenberg, E., and Wersäll, J.: Morphological changes in vestibular hair cells in a strain of the waltzing guinea pig. Acta oto-lar. *67:* 521–534 (1969).

3   Flock, Å.: Physiological properties of sensory hairs in the ear; in Psychophysics and physiology of hearing, pp. 15–26 (Academic Press, New York 1977).

4   Flock, Å. and Cheung, H.: Actin filaments in sensory hairs of the inner ear receptor cells. J. Cell Biol. *75:* 339–343 (1977).

5   Hitchcock, S.E.: Regulation of motility in nonmuscle cells. J. Cell Biol. *74:* 1–15 (1977).

6   Ibsen, L.H. and Risty, T.K.: A new character in guinea pigs, waltzing. Anat. Rec. *44:* 294 (1929).

7   Isenberg, G. and Wohlfarth-Botterman, K.E.: Transformation of cytoplasmic actin. Cell Tiss. Res. *173:* 495–528 (1976).

8   Ishikawa, H.; Bischoff, R., and Holtzer, H.: Formation of arrowhead complexes with heavy meromyosin in a variety of cell types. J. Cell Biol. *43:* 312–327 (1969).

9   Lurie, M.H.: The waltzing (circling) guinea pig. Am. Otol. *50:* 113 (1941).
10   Margossian, S.S. and Lowey, S.: Structure of the myosin molecule. IV. Interaction of myosin and its subfragments with adenosine triphosphate and f-actin. J. molec. Biol. *74:* 313–330 (1973).
11   Maupin-Szamier, P. and Pollard, T.D.: Actin filament destruction by osmium tetroxide. J. Cell Biol. *77:* 837–852 (1978).
12   Simionescu, N. and Simionescu, M.: Galloylglucoses of low molecular weight as a mordant in electron microscopy I. Procedure and evidence for mordanting effect. J. Cell Biol. *70:* 608–621 (1976).
13   Taylor, D.L.; Condeelis, J.S.; Moore, P.L., and Allen, R.D.: The contractile basis of ameboid movement. I. The chemical control of motility in isolated cytoplasm. J. Cell Biol. *59:* 378–394 (1973).
14   Tilney, L.G.: Actin filaments in the acrosomal reaction of *Limulus* sperm. J. Cell Biol. *64:* 289–310 (1975).
15   Tilney, L.G.: The polymerization of actin. II. How non-filamentous actin becomes non-randomly distributed in sperm: evidence for the association of this actin with membranes. J. Cell Biol. *69:* 51–72 (1976).
16   Wersäll, J.: Studies on the structure and innervation of the sensory epithelium of the cristae ampullares in the guinea pig. Acta oto-lar. *126:* suppl., pp. 1–85 (1956).

Å. Flock, MD, Fysiologiska Institutionen II, Karolinska Institutet,
Solnavägen 1, S-104 01 Stockholm (Sweden)

stimulation levels (up to 100 dB) the function of melanin would be in auditory adaptation and at higher levels (120 dB) it would be in auditory fatigue. They therefore postulated that melanin might have a protective effect at high-noise levels.

With knowledge of the physico-chemical properties of melanin, the idea that it may be involved in the hearing process has been put forward [17]. As seen from the above review of the literature, findings have been made that may imply that hyperpigmentation has a positive impact and pigment deficiency a negative impact on hearing. In the light of these observations we consider that the possible role of melanin in the hearing and balance functions should be discussed and analysed further.

Melanin can be regarded as an amorphous semiconductor and has a high redox potential. The electronic properties of the melanins are probably best explained in terms of the amorphous semiconductor theory [12, 13] in which electronic states are closely coupled to vibrational modes of the polymer. Theoretically, with these properties melanin might participate in different processes in the internal ear [17]. Thus, (1) it could act as an energy transformer, e.g. transforming mechanical to electrical energy, and (2) it could have a protective effect in that the sound energy peaks could be cut off through exitation of the melanin, with subsequent reversion to the resting state during emission of thermal energy (fig.2).

The two postulated properties of melanin, energy transfer and sound protection, may be altered by substances with melanin affinity. Both a beneficial and a noxious effect of substances with melanin affinity therefore have to be considered.

Summary

The capacity of the melanin in the internal ear to accumulate and retain labelled lidocaine, bupivacaine and chlorpromazine after intravenous and intraperitoneal injection was examined by whole-body autoradiography. Both young pigmented hooded rats and albino rats were studied. In the pigmented rats chlorpromazine showed the greatest accumulation, which was more pronounced in the cochlea than in the vestibular portion. The other two substances were evenly distributed in the internal ear. After a single injection of chlorpromazine and of bupivacaine these substances were still bound to the melanin of the internal ear after 14 days, which was the longest survival time. Lidocaine, on the other hand, had disappeared after only 4 days. In albino animals there was very weak, transient uptake of chlorpromazine and bupivacaine, but not of lidocaine, in the internal ear. In studies *in vitro* on isolated bovine eye melanin there was considerably greater adsorption of chlorpromazine than of lidocaine and bupivacaine.

References

1   Beck, C.: Das Pigment der Stria vascularis. Arch. Ohr.- Nas.- KehlkHeilk./Z. Hals- Nasen- Ohrenheilk. *179:* 51 (1961).
2   Bonaccorsi, P.: Il colore dell'iride come 'Test' di valutazione quantitativa, nell'uomo, della concentrazzione di melanina nella stria vascolare. Annali Lar. Otol. Rinol. Faring. *64:* 725 (1965).
3   Dencker, L. and Lindquist, N.G.: Distribution of labelled chloroquine in the inner ear. Archs Otolar. *101:* 185 (1975).
4   Englesson, S.; Larsson, B.; Lyttkens, L.; Lindquist, N.G., and Stahle, J.: Accumulation of ^{14}C-lidocaine in the inner ear. Acta oto-lar. *82:* 297 (1976).
5   Hilding, D.A. and Ginzburg, R.D.: Pigmentation of the stria vascularis. Acta oto-lar. *84:* 24 (1977).
6   Hood, J.D.; Poole, J.P., and Freedman, L.: The influence of eye colour upon temporary threshold shift. Audiology *15:* 449 (1976).
7   Karsai, L.K.; Bergman, M., and Choo, Y.B.: Hearing in ethnically different longshorement. Archs Oto-lar. *96:* 499 (1972).
8   La Ferriere, K.A.; Arenberg, I.K.; Hawkins, J.E., and Johnsson, L.G.: Melanocytes of the vestibular labyrinth and their relationship to the microvasculature. Ann. Otol Rhinol. Lar. *83:* 685 (1974).
9   Lindquist, N.G.: Accumulation of drugs on melanin. Acta Radiol., suppl. 325, p. 1 (1973).
10 Lindquist, N.G. and Ullberg, S.: The melanin affinity of chloroquine and chlorpromazine studied by whole body autoradiography. Acta pharmac. tox., suppl. 2, p. 1 (1972).
11 Lyttkens, L.; Larsson, B.; Göller, H.; Englesson, S., and Stahle, J.: Melanin capacity to accumulate drugs in the internal ear. Acta oto-lar. (in press 1978).
12 McGinness, J. and Proctor, P.: The importance of the fact that melanin is black. J. theor. Biol. *39:* 677 (1973).
13 McGinness, J.; Corry, P., and Proctor, P.: Amorphous semiconductor switching in melanins. Science *183:* 853 (1974).
14 Melding, P.S.; Goodey, R.J., and Thorne, P.R.: The use of intravenous lignocaine in the diagnosis and treatment of tinnitus. J. Lar. Otol. *92:* 115 (1978).
15 Post, R.H.: Hearing acquity variation among negroes and whites. Eugen. Q. *11:* 65 (1964).
16 Potts, A.M.: The reaction of uveal pigment *in vitro* with polycylic compounds. Investve Ophthal. *3:* 405 (1964).
17 Proctor, P.; McGinness, J., and Corry, P.: A hypothesis on the preferential destruction of melanized tissues. J. theor. Biol. *48:* 19 (1974).
18 Roberts, J. and Bayliss, P.: Hearing levels of adults by race, region and area of residence; in Vital and health statistics. Data from the National Health Survey. National Center for Health Statistics, Series 11, No. 26 (1967).
19 Savin, C.: The blood vessels and pigmentary cells of the inner ear. Ann. Otol. Rhinol. Lar. *74:* 611 (1965).
20 Sieber, J. und Schmidt, H.: Histologische und histochemische Untersuchungen an häutigen Bogengängen. Z. Lar. Rhinol. Otol. *41:* 46 (1962).

21   Tota, G. and Bocci, G.: L'imporanza del colore dell'iride nella valutazione della resistenza dell'udito all'affaticamento. Rev. Oto-neuro-oftal. *42:* 183 (1967).

22   Ullberg, S.: Studies on the distribution and fate of S^{35}-labelled benzylpenicillin in the body. Acta radiol., suppl. 118, p. 1 (1954).

23   Ullberg, S.: The technique of whole body autoradiography. Cryosectioning of large specimens. Science Tools, The LKB Instrumental Journal, Special issue, p 2. LKB-produkter AB, S-161 25 Bromma 1, Sweden (1977).

24   Ullberg, S.; Lindquist, N.G., and Sjöstrand, S.E.: Accumulation of chorio-retino-toxic drugs in the foetal eye. Nature, Lond. *227:* 1257 (1970).

25   Wolff, D.: Melanin in the inner ear. Archs Otolar. *14:* 195 (1931).

Leif Lyttkens, MD, Department of Otolaryngology, University Hospital,
S-750 14 Uppsala (Sweden)

Adv. Oto-Rhino-Laryng., vol. 25, pp. 26–33 (Karger, Basel 1979)

Calcium Ion Uptake and Exchange in Otoconia

M.D. Ross

Department of Anatomy, University of Michigan, Ann Arbor, Mich.

Introduction

The otoconia of higher vertebrates are crystals of calcite [*Carlström et al.*, 1953; *Carlström and Engström*, 1955] containing a small amount of organic material. They are found in or on the otolithic membranes of the saccular and utricular maculas and act as weight-lending structures, making the membranes more responsive to forces of linear acceleration.

It would seem to be incorrect, however, to look no farther than the weight-lending capacity of the otoconia in considering the possible importance of these crystals to the economy of the inner ear. To do so would be to ignore their most central features: that otoconia are highly ordered mineral/organic material deposits existing in a fluid medium and, as such, must be constantly interacting ionically with their environment.

In order to begin to understand what these ionic interactions might mean to inner ear function it seemed plausible to consider those of another complex mineral deposit of the body, the skeleton. It is well known that aside from its supportive function, the skeleton serves as a means of rapidly removing excess calcium ions from the blood and storing them until they are needed once again. But the skeleton functions not only in calcium ion homeostasis, but also stores and releases phosphate (and carbonate) ions, thereby contributing greatly to the buffering capacity of the blood against acidic substances. Otoconia might serve the endolymph of the inner ear in these same ways: as a means of removing excess calcium from endolymph; as a repository of these ions against future need; and as a storage site for carbonate ions to insure the buffering capacity of the endolymph.

It also seemed possible that, although the basic functions of the saccular and utricular otoconia were likely identical, the demands placed upon the two kinds of otoconia for ion interactions were not. This inference was drawn partly from work which showed that saccular and utricular otoconia differed in their potential for postnatal growth and in their proneness to age-related demineralization [*Johnsson* 1971; *Johnsson and Hawkins,* 1972; *Ross et al.,* 1976], and partly from the work of *Sellick and Johnstone* [1972] and *Sellick et al.* [1972] which indicated that saccular and utricular endolymph were not identical ionically.

A series of experiments was designed, therefore, to study saccular and utricular otoconia as dynamic mineral deposits by comparing their uptake of ⁴⁵Ca to that of bone, utilizing the sensitive method of liquid scintillation spectrometry. Radioisotope methods have been applied to otoconia previously [*Belanger,* 1960; *Veenhof,* 1969; *Preston et al.,* 1975] but with mixed results. Only *Preston et al.* [1975], using liquid scintillation spectrometry, were able to show ⁴⁵Ca uptake into otolithic membranes of adult animals (gerbils) 24 h after a single dose, with some retention of radioactivity for up to 27 days. If otoconia are dynamic structures, however, constantly interacting with their environment as does bone, then substantial uptake of the tracer should take place shortly after injection. *Bronner* [1958] demonstrated that 85% of a ⁴⁵Ca dose had entered the rat skeleton by 4 h.

This report deals, then, with the results of four experiments covering primarily the first 2–24 h after a single injection of ⁴⁵Ca into young adult rats, although some shorter and longer survival times are included. Work is still in progress, but findings are interpreted in a preliminary way in light of the hypotheses tested: that otoconia are dynamic mineral deposits; and that saccular and utricular otoconia function in slightly different milieus and could have different patterns or levels of calcium ion uptake.

Material and Methods

150 young adult (210–490 g) Sprague-Dawley male and female rats were injected with ⁴⁵Ca (4 mCi/kg body weight, *Preston et al.* [1975]). Postinjection survival times were 5 min to 7 days. The anesthetized animals were sacrificed by exsanguination while being perfused with physiological saline to reduce possible contamination of the samples by blood-borne ⁴⁵Ca during collection. Fresh otolithic membranes were microdissected under several changes of 70% alcohol. Some otoconia were inevitably lost, but all later measurements of radioactivity were interpreted on a weight basis to compensate for this.

Saccular and utricular otoconia were pooled separately, by pairs in the first experiment, and from 6 animals in the rest. In the fourth experiment, otoconia were separated by sex as well as by macular origin. All otoconial samples were treated similarly. They

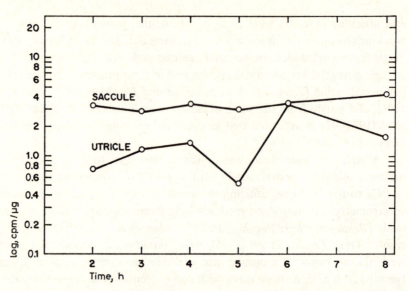

Fig. 1. This graph compares saccular and utricular ⁴⁵Ca uptake in Experiment 2. Each point on the graph represents cpm/µg obtained from otoconia pooled from 6 animals.

were collectedviously we on preighed foils, dried (110°C) to drive off bound water, then weighed (Cahn electrobalance), dissolved in 1 *N* HCl and subjected to ordinary procedures for liquid scintillation spectrometry.

Blood samples were taken at 15 and 30 min, at 1, 2, and 4 h, and at sacrifice in experiments lasting 4 h or more. For shorter times, blood was collected according to schedule up to sacrifice. The blood samples (<2 ml) were allowed to clot, then centrifuged, and 20 µl aliquots of the supernatant serum were prepared for scintillation counting.

Bone chips (femur and otic capsule) were taken at sacrifice, scraped, washed, and then prepared individually according to procedures used for otoconia. In the fourth experiment, a total of 48 femur, 24 otic bone, and 60 blood samples were analyzed for the single survival time tested (4 h).

Measurements of radioactivity were determined on the basis of counts per minute/ microgram dry weight (cpm/µg) for each mineral, and counts per minute/per milliliter (cpm/ml) for serum.

Results

The average weight of the paired saccular otoconial masses in the first experiment was 9 µg, while the utricular masses averaged 14.5 µg (24 samples in each case). ⁴⁵Ca uptake by this quantity of otoconia during shorter survival times (up to 2 h) was not sufficient for collection of reliable data.

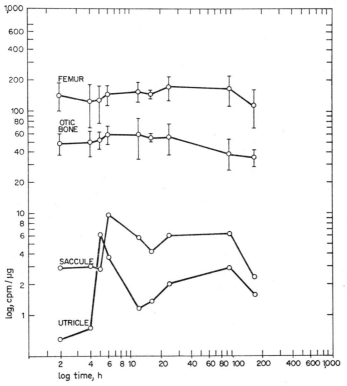

Fig. 2. ^{45}Ca uptake by saccular and utricular otoconia is compared to that of femur and otic bone in this graph. The data were obtained from Experiment 3 and are expressed in cpm/µg. Otoconia values represent counts obtained from pooled samples (6 animals). Each bone value represents an average of the counts obtained from 6 individual samples; 95% confidence intervals are indicated by the bars.

The findings did indicate, however, that measurable ^{45}Ca occurred by 2 h and suggested that saccular and utricular otoconia interacted with the tracer to different extents. The first experiment, then, provided the basis for the others that followed, in which otoconia from 6 animals were pooled to increase the level of radioactivity.

The second and third experiments were designed to examine survival times between 2 h and 1 week. Saccular otoconia continued to show a higher level of uptake of ^{45}Ca than utricular otoconia (fig. 1, 2). Otoconia from both maculas demonstrated appreciable levels of ^{45}Ca (as did bone mineral) at times when the level of the radioisotope had fallen considerably in the serum. Serum ^{45}Ca peaked within 30 min.

Otoconial ^{45}Ca uptake followed the general pattern of incorporation of radioactive calcium into bone mineral (fig. 2), although the latter occurred on a scale 10–100 times greater in magnitude. In these experiments, ^{45}Ca levels were always higher in the femur than in otic bone (fig. 2).

Data from the third experiment showed that females often demonstrated higher levels of ^{45}Ca in serum and lower levels of radioactivity in the bone samples than did males, especially during the first several hours after injection, although these differences became less pronounced at 1 week. A fourth experiment was designed, therefore, to test these trends further and to look for possible sex-related differences in otoconial uptake that might provide a basis for further investigation. One survival time, 4 h, was selected because of the high level of radioactivity evident at this time. The results of experiment 4 continued to show differences in ^{45}Ca uptake into bone mineral in males and females at this time point. The data were found to be statistically significant (at the $\alpha = 0.02$ level) in the case of the femur. The number of bone samples at other time points is still too small for such analysis. The differences in male-female otoconial ^{45}Ca uptake at 4 h were (in cpm/µg) 6.5–4.1 for the saccule and 2.1–1.5 for the utricle. The statistical significance of this single finding cannot be determined.

Discussion

The results of these experiments indicate that otoconia are dynamic structures which take up ^{45}Ca on a time scale generally comparable to that of bone but to a much lesser degree, with saccular otoconia taking up more ^{45}Ca than utricular otoconia under identical experimental conditions. Aside from these observations, no further meaning can be attached to the various peaks and troughs shown for otoconial ^{45}Ca uptake. This is because each point represents but a single sample for the times tested, and the significance of the final decline in radioactivity between 4 and 7 days cannot be assessed without following the ^{45}Ca over longer survival times. Thus, current results do not allow a differentiation to be made between relatively short-term ion uptake and exchange that could involve organic material alone, and possible long-term incorporation of the ^{45}Ca into the otoconial crystal lattices. Further work is in progress to elucidate this issue.

Although many factors influence the actual level of uptake of tracer substance by bone or by otoconia, not the least of these are the comparable sizes of the two kinds of crystals involved, the biological activity of the organic fractions of the minerals, and the dynamics of the fluids in which the mineral complexes are immersed. Otoconia are enormous in size compared to the hydroxyapatite crystals of bone mineral, and the surface areas available for ion interactions are inversely proportional. With respect to the organic portion of the otoconia, neither its size, chemical composition (and ability to adsorb calcium ions), or precise physical arrangement in the crystals is known. The turnover rate of endolymph is equally obscure.

The possibility that a sex-related factor may influence ^{45}Ca uptake in the labyrinth as well as in the skeleton is presented for its obvious clinical interest. Much more research will be necessary to confirm or refute this observation. That 'bone calcium entry' varies with sex (and age) has been reported previously [Bronner, 1973]. Preston et al. [1975] founnd an apparent sex-related difference in ^{45}Ca uptake into bone mineral in the gerbil; their findings could not be evaluated further because the male and female animals came from different suppliers. Animals used in the present study came from the same supplier and the males and females were of approximately equivalent age and sexual development. Their weights varied, however, and the possibility that a dose-dependent factor was operative cannot be excluded at this time.

The finding that saccular and utricular otoconia differ in ^{45}Ca uptake in the rat has not been reported previously but fits well with numerous prior results which indicate that the fluid environments of otoconia from the two maculas are not identical. Sellick and Johnstone [1972] and Sellick et al. [1972] have provided evidence that saccular endolymph resembles cochlear endolymph more than utricular with respect to sodium ion concentration. They have suggested that the saccule may depend upon the cochlea for both its endolymph and its weak electrical potential. Kimura [1969] has found that dark cells, thought to be important in endolymph production, are lacking in the saccule of the guinea pig, although species differences may exist [Smith, 1970]. Bast [1928] and many others have described a utriculoendolymphatic valve which appears to guard the utricular outlet into the endolymphatic duct; but the saccular and cochlear endolymph are confluent through the ductus reuniens.

These and many other lines of evidence suggest that the fluid environments of the superior and inferior portions of the labyrinth have become more restricted with phylogeny. It is possible, then, that saccular otoconia help preserve the ionic homeostasis of the inferior part of the labyrinth, which includes the cochlea, while the utricular otoconia perform this same function for the superior part, which includes the semicircular canals. Such concepts, if supported by further research, would lend great significance to calcium and carbonate ions in the general economy of the inner ear, but these are the only two ions stored in any quantity in the entire labyrinth and they are stored in the calcite of the otoconia.

Summary

Calcium ion uptake into otoconia and bone mineral of the young adult rat was studied by use of ^{45}Ca and liquid scintillation spectrometry. Results showed that saccular and utricular otoconia take up ^{45}Ca in a time course generally comparable to bone but on a much lower scale. Saccular otoconia showed greater uptake than utricular. The results are interpreted to indicate the dynamic nature of saccular and utricular otoconia and their possible importance in preserving ionic homeostasis of the inferior and superior parts of the labyrinth, respectively.

Acknowledgements

This research was supported by NASA Grant NSG 9047. I thank Dr. *D. Dziewiatowski* for his encouragement and guidance in early stages of this work, and Miss *Iris Mechigian* and Mr. *Thomas Williams* for their technical assistance. I also thank Dr. *Jochen Schacht* and Dr. *Donald Peacor* for their comments during preparation of the manuscript.

References

Bast, T.H.: The utriculo-endolymphatic valve. Anat. Rec. *40:* 61–65 (1928).
Belanger, L.F.: Development, structure and composition of the otolithic organs of the rat; in Sognnaes, Calcification in biological systems, pp. 151–162 Am. Ass. Adv. Sci. Publ. No. 64, Washington 1960.
Bronner, F.: Disposition of intraperitoneally injected calcium-45 in suckling rats. J. gen. Physiol. *41:* 767–782 (1958).
Bronner, F.: Kinetic and cybernetic analysis of calcium metabolism; in Irving, Calcium and phosphorus metabolism, pp. 149–186 (Academic Press, New York 1973).
Carlström, D. and Engström, H.: The ultrastructure of statoconia. Acta oto-lar. *45:* 14–18 (1955).
Carlström, D.; Engström, H., and Hjorth, S.: Electron microscopic and x-ray diffraction studies of statoconia. Laryngoscope *63:* 1052–1057 (1953).
Johnsson, L.G.: Degenerative changes and anomalies of the vestibular system in man. Laryngoscope *81:* 1682–1694 (1971).

Johnsson, L.G. and Hawkins, J.E., jr.: Sensory and neural degeneration with aging, as seen in microdissections of the human inner ear. Ann. Otol. Rhinol. Lar. *81:* 179–193 (1972).

Kimura, R.S.: Distribution, structure, and function of dark cells in the vestibular labyrinth. Ann. Otol. Rhinol. Lar. *78:* 542–561 (1969).

Preston, R.E.; Johnsson, L.G.; Hill, J.H., and Schacht, J.: Incorporation of radioactive calcium into otolithic membranes and middle ear ossicles of the gerbil. Acta otolar. *80:* 269–275 (1975).

Ross, M.D.; Peacor, D.; Johnsson, L.G., and Allard, L.F.: Observations on normal and degenerating human otoconia. Ann. Otol. Rhinol. Lar. *85:* 310–326 (1976).

Sellick, P.M. and Johnstone, B.M.: Changes in cochlear endolymph Na$^+$ concentration measured with Na$^+$ specific microelectrodes. Pflügers Arch. ges. Physiol. *336:* 11–20 (1972).

Sellick, P.M. and Johnstone, B.M.: The electrophysiology of the saccule. Pflügers Arch. ges. Physiol. *336:* 28–34 (1972).

Sellick, P.M.; Johnstone, J.R., and Johnstone, B.M.: The electrophysiology of the utricle. Pflügers Arch. ges. Physiol. *336:* 21–27 (1972).

Smith, C.A.: The extrasensory cells of the vestibule; in Paparella, Biochemical mechanisms in hearing and deafness, pp. 171–185 (Thomas, Springfield 1970).

Veenhof, V.B.: The development of statoconia in mice. Akad. Wetensch. Amsterdam Verh., 2° reeks: *58:* 1–49 (1969).

M.D. Ross, PhD, Department of Anatomy, University of Michigan,
Ann Arbor, MI 48109 (USA)

Adv. Oto-Rhino-Laryng., vol. 25, pp. 34–40 (Karger, Basel 1979)

Anatomy of the Para-Vestibular Canaliculus[1]

I. Sando and T. Egami[2]

Eye and Ear Hospital of Pittsburgh, Department of Otolaryngology and Pathology, University of Pittsburgh School of Medicine, Pittsburgh, Pa. and Department of Otolaryngology, University of Colorado School of Medicine, Denver, Colo.

Introduction

Siebenmann [1894] reported that the canalis accessorius aqueductus vestibuli is a separate canal from the vestibular aqueduct (VA) and he indicated that it contains veins from the utricle and the semicircular canal ends. However, he did not specifically describe the entire course of this canal. Recently, *Ogura and Clemis* [1971], termed this canal the para-vestibular canaliculus (PVC) and, mainly using a technique of microdissection with osmic acid stain, described its course in detail. As part of their description, they mentioned that the PVC contains both an artery and a vein. Later, *Stahle and Wilbrand* [1974] confirmed these findings by much the same technique and reported additional anatomical information such as the proximal branching of the PVC and the distal branching of the artery of the PVC. The purpose of this study is to define further and to analyze the course and contents of this important anatomical structure through an examination of serial histologic sections which have been stained by various methods.

[1] Supported by research grants NS 09203 and NS 13787 from the National Institute of Neurological and Communicative Diseases and Strokes, USA.

[2] The authors express their appreciation to *Kenneth M. Grundfast*, MD, *Susumu Suehiro*, MD, *Takehiko Harada*, MD, *Pamela Marks, Shelly Frish, Cheryl Mervis, Roxanne Libby*, and *Audrey Zatorsky* for their assistance.

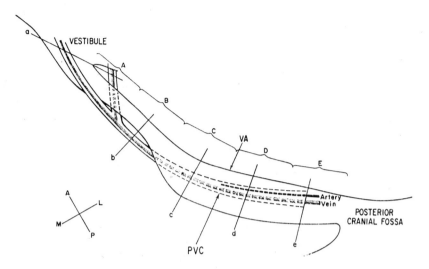

Fig. 1. Schematic drawing of the PVC and its vascular contents (vein and artery) along with the VA in a right temporal bone in a 'bird's-eye view', demonstrates the most common course of the PVC. A, B, C, D and E indicate vestibular orifice area, isthmus area, proximal rugose area, intermediate area and cranial orifice area of the VA for orientation in tracing the PVC. a, b, c, d and e are vestibular orifice portion, isthmus portion, proximal rugose portion, intermediate portion and aqueductal orifice portion of the PVC to measure the size of the PVC itself and its vascular contents. A = Anterior; L = lateral; M = medial; P = posterior.

Materials and Methods

20 temporal bones from 20 cadavers with no history of any congenital anomaly or otologic disease were fixed in 10% formalin solution, decalcified in 1% nitric acid solution, embedded in celloidin, and sectioned horizontally at intervals of 20 μm. Every tenth section was routinely stained with hematoxylin and eosin (HE) and, when necessary to delineate further the course of the PVC or its contents, additional sections were stained with HE and examined. To identify arteries and veins, some of the sections not stained with HE were stained either by Verhoeff-Van Gieson's method or by Mallory's method.

With a light microscope, the relationship was examined between the location of the PVC and the following five areas of the VA (fig. 1): (A) Vestibular orifice area – VA between the vestibular orifice of the endolymphatic duct and the isthmus part of the endolymphatic duct. (B) Isthmus area – VA adjacent to the isthmus part of the endolymphatic duct. (C) Proximal rugose area – V γadjacent to the most proximal rugose part of the endolymphatic sac. (D) Intermediate area – VA between the proximal rugose area (C) and the cranial orifice area (E). (E) Cranial orifice area – VA adjacent to the cranial orifice for the endolymphatic sac.

Measurements were made of the diameter of the PVC itself, and of the largest vein and artery, if any, within the PVC for five selected portions of the PVC.

These selected portions were: (a) Vestibular orifice portion – PVC adjacent to the vestibular orifice of the VA. (b) Isthmus portion – PVC adjacent to the center portion of the isthmus area (B) of the VA. (c) Proximal rugose portion – PVC adjacent to the center portion of the proximal rugose area (C) of the VA. (d) Intermediate portion – PVC midway between the proximal rugose portion (c) and the aqueductal orifice portion (e). (e) Aqueductal orifice portion – PVC where the VA and PVC merge, or where the PVC enters the posterior cranial fossa (PCF).

Findings

Course of the PVC

The usual course of the PVC was found to be as follows: the PVC originated at the vestibule as two canaliculi, one superior and one inferolateral to the vestibular orifice area of the VA (15 specimens). These two canaliculi merged into a single canal which ran either medially or inferomedially to the isthmus area of the VA (10 specimens). The PVC was usually located inferior to the proximal rugose area of the VA (15 specimens) and either inferior (7 specimens) or inferolateral (5 specimens) to the intermediate area of the VA. The PVC was found to merge into the inferior region of the cranial orifice area of the VA in 8 specimens. Of those 8 specimens, 4 specimens showed the PVC merging into the inferolateral region of the VA. The distance between the point of merger of the PVC with the VA and the cranial orifice of the VA could be measured in all 8 specimens, and was 1.99 mm on the average (it ranged between 0.7 and 2.9 mm).

Variations in the course of the PVC were observed. In the vestibular orifice area (A) of the VA, a single PVC was present superior to the VA in 4 specimens. Also in area (A), 2 specimens had two PVCs present and located either superior to the VA (1 specimen) or merging into the superior region and the inferolateral region of the VA, resulting in no PVC observed distal to this area (1 specimen). In the isthmus area (B) of the VA, two PVCs were still present in the areas medial and inferior to the VA (4 specimens), lateral and inferior to the VA (1 specimen), and medial to the VA and close to each other (1 specimen). Also in area (B), in the other 3 specimens, a single PVC was located either lateral (2 specimens) or inferolateral (1 specimen) to the VA. In the proximal rugose area (C) of the VA, two PVCs were still observed to be close together in the areas inferior

(1 specimen), inferolateral (1 specimen), and inferomedial (1 specimen) to the VA. Also in area (C) in the other specimen, a single PVC was present in the area inferomedial to the VA. In the intermediate area (D) of the VA, a single PVC was found to merge into the inferior region of the VA (4 specimens), or observed to have a course inferomedial to the VA (1 specimen). In this area, two PVCs, one merging into the inferior region of the VA and one located inferior to the VA, were observed in 1 specimen. Also observed was the disappearance of the PVC in the otic capsule in 1 specimen which had another PVC merging into the inferior region of the VA in this area. In the cranial orifice area (E) of the VA, a single PVC was still seen separately from the VA in the area either inferolateral (3 specimens) or inferior (2 specimens) to the VA. In the former 3 specimens, the merging point of the PVC directly to the PCF was observed in the area, 0.7–1.5 mm posterior to the inferolateral region of the cranial orifice area of the VA. In the latter 2 specimens, the merging point could be observed also in the PCF as being located posteroinferior to the most inferior region of the cranial orifice area of the VA, but no measurement could be made of the distance from the cranial orifice of the VA to the point of merger due to the fact that different sectioning angles had been used for the merging point of the PVC and for the cranial orifice area of the VA. Disappearance of the PVC in the otic capsule was noted in 1 specimen which carried a single PVC from the vestibular orifice area to the intermediate area of the VA.

Size and Contents of the PVC

The average diameters of the PVC at its vestibular orifice portion and at its isthmus portion were 95 and 94 μm, respectively. As the PVC coursed toward the PCF, the diameter widened to averages of 125, 158, 206 μm at the proximal rugose portion, the intermediate portion, and the aqueductal orifice portion, respectively.

The PVC contained a large vein with an average diameter of 35 μm throughout its course in all specimens. The average diameters of the lumen of the vein in five representative portions of the PVC (the vestibular orifice portion, the isthmus portion, the proximal rugose portion, the intermediate portion, and the aqueductal orifice portion) were 47, 51, 60, 55, and 53 μm, respectively. It was 58 μm, average, outside of the PVC where the vein exited from the PVC to either the VA or the PCF. In addition, the PVC contained small veins and capillaries particularly in its posterior cranial portion. It was also found that, as the PVC coursed toward the VA, more perivascular dense connective tissue was observed in the VA.

Small arteries were present only in the posterior cranial portion of the PVC in 13 specimens (65%). In the remaining 7 specimens (35%), there were no arteries observed throughout the course of the PVC. The major artery of the PVC was smaller in the intermediate portion than in the aqueductal orifice portion of the PVC. There was no artery in its own bony channel coursing from the PVC through the otic capsule to the VA or vice versa, although the capillaries in the minute bony canaliculi were noted to surround and to communicate with the PVC, the VA, or both. In one specimen, however, there were small arteries and veins which exited from the aqueductal orifice portion of the PVC and, housed in separate bony canaliculi, disappeared with their canaliculi into the otic capsule, in the area near the cranial orifice area of the VA.

Discussion

The size of the PVC as measured in this study (0.094–0.206 mm) is similar to those reported by *Ogura and Clemis* [1971] (0.1–0.3 mm) and *Stahle and Wilbrand* [1974] (0.1–0.2 mm). Further, in this study it was found that the PVC is larger at the aqueduct orifice portion than at the vestibular orifice portion.

The course of the midportion of the PVC in this study was similar to that previously reported by *Ogura and Clemis* [1971] and *Stahle and Wilbrand* [1974]. The observation in this study that 16 specimens (80%) had two separate PVCs near the vestibule confirms a similar finding reported by *Stahle and Wilbrand* [1974]. However, it appears that the existence of two PVCs in this area was more commonly seen in the specimens examined in this study than in those examined by *Stahle and Wilbrand* [1974]. At the other end of the PVC, near the cranial orifice area, or the intermediate area of the VA in 14 specimens (70%) it could be seen that the VA and the PVC merged to form a common channel; this appears to be a higher incidence of merging of the VA and the PVC than had been found by *Stahle and Wilbrand* [1974]. *Stahle and Wilbrand* [1974] reported that the PVC and its contained artery sometimes split into several branches distally. In contrast, in this study only 1 of the 20 specimens had distal branches which contained artery and vein. When they were followed in serial sections, it could be seen that the branches became progressively smaller in size, then ended within the otic capsule.

The vascular contents of the PVC as observed in this study are notable. *Stahle and Wilbrand* [1974] mentioned that the endolymphatic sac receives a dual blood supply, one from the posterior meningeal artery, and a substantial supply from the vestibular branch of the labyrinthine artery through the artery of the PVC. In this study, the observed locations of the arteries within the PVC relative to the location of the endolymphatic sac seem to indicate that most of the arterial blood supply to the endolymphatic sac must come from the posterior meningeal artery.

In 13 (65%) of the specimens arteries could be identified only in the portion of the PVC near the PCF and in the other 7 (35%) specimens no arteries were seen in the PVC. Also, there was no artery observed in a separate bony channel coursing through the otic capsule and forming a communication between the VA and the PVC. In none of the 20 specimens examined could arteries be seen within the vestibular end of the PVC. Thus, it appears that any arteries contained in the PVC near the cranial orifice area of the VA (in proximity to the endolymphatic sac) area probably branches of the artery of the VA or branches of the posterior meningeal artery. This is consistent with the description by *Bast and Anson* [1949] of a branch of the posterior meningeal artery supplying the wall of the endolymphatic sac. Most likely, the arteries seen in the PVC supply blood to the contents of the PVC and perhaps to some of the surrounding otic capsule rather than to the VA or the endolymphatic sac.

Since a large vein was always observed throughout the entire length of the PVC, it appears that the PVC contains the main venous drainage system from the vestibule, as was earlier described by *Siebenmann* [1894].

Summary

A histologic study of the para-vestibular canaliculus (PVC), its contents, and its relationship to the vestibular aqueduct (VA), is presented. 20 normal human temporal bones were fixed in 10% formalin solution, embedded in celloidin, and sectioned horizontally at intervals of 20 μm. Every tenth section was stained with hematoxylin and eosin (HE) and studied under a light microscope. Three significant observations were made. First, in 80% of the specimens, two rather than one PVC were found in the area of the vestibular orifice of the VA. Second, in 70% of the specimens, the PVC was found to merge with the VA rather than to enter the posterior cranial fossa (PCF) separately. Third, in all the specimens examined, a vein was seen to traverse the entire length of the PVC. However, in 17 specimens, no artery could be identified within the PVC. In the 13 (65%) specimens in which arteries could be identified in the PVC, the arteries extended only half the length of the PVC, from the PCF to the VA. In no specimen examined could arteries be seen extending the full length of the PVC from the PCF to the vestibule.

References

Bast, T.H. and Anson, B.J.: Blood supply of the otic capsule; in The temporal bone and ear, pp. 249–261 (Thomas, Springfield 1949).

Ogura, Y. and Clemis, J.: A study of the gross anatomy of the human vestibular aqueduct. Ann. Otolar. *80:* 813–825 (1971).

Siebenmann, F.: Die Gefässe des Labyrinthes; in die Blut-Gefässe im Labyrinthe des menschlichen Ohres, pp. 10–29 (Bergmann, Wiesbaden 1894).

Stahle, J. and Wilbrand, H.: The para-vestibular canaliculus. Am. J. Otolar. *3:* 262–270 (1974).

I. Sando, MD, Department of Otolaryngology and Pathology,
University of Pittsburgh, School of Medicine, 3500 Terrace Street,
Pittsburgh, PA 15216 (USA)

Adv. Oto-Rhino-Laryng., vol. 25, pp. 41–48 (Karger, Basel 1979)

The Cochlear Blood Flow in Relation to Noise and Cervical Sympathectomy[1]

C. Angelborg, E. Hultcrantz and M. Beausang-Linder[2]

Department of Otolaryngology, University Hospital, and the Institute of
Physiology and Medical Biophysics, Biomedical Centre, University of Uppsala,
Uppsala

Introduction

The precise way in which noise damages the inner ear, temporarily
and permanently, is still not clear but this field of research is becoming
increasingly important with regard to prophylactics and treatment of noise-
induced hearing loss.

In other organs than the ear, for instance, in the tail of the rat [4],
noise has been shown to reduce the blood flow and exposure to noise has
also been demonstrated to reduce endolymphatic oxygen tension [12, 15].
Thus it lies close at hand to suspect that noise causes vasoconstriction also
in the inner ear and that this might be a contributory mechanism behind
sensory cell damage in the cochlea. Such a vasoconstriction might be caused
via the adrenergic nervous system but this question has yet to be answered.
The so-called microsphere method has been adapted for blood flow studies
in the cochlea [2] and the method successfully used to investigate the effect
of sympathetic stimulation on the cochlear blood circulation [7]. The same
method was applied in the present investigation to study the reactions of
the cochlear blood circulation upon noise exposure and to examine whether
cervical sympathectomy will influence the cochlear blood flow under these

[1] This work was supported by the Swedish Medical Research Council (project No.
B78-17X-04782-03 and B78-14X-00147-14B) and 'Tysta Skolan'.
[2] The authors are indebted to *Alf Svedberg* PhD for technical assistance and for
help with the statistical analysis.

experimental conditions. Moreover, different forms of anesthetics were used to study if and how the type of anesthesia might influence the results.

Material and Method

15 cats of both sexes, weighing between 2.4 and 3.6 kg, were used. 5 animals were anesthetized by ketamine-chloride 30 mg/kg bodyweight i.m. and 10 by chloroform initially, followed by i.v. administration of chloralose 75 mg/kg body weight.

The cats were tracheotomized and ventilated by a Palmer pump. Catheters were inserted into both femoral arteries, one for blood pressure measurements and the other for blood sampling. The cervical sympathetic trunk was exposed on one side and transected at the level of the upper cervical ganglion. The vagal nerve was left intact. The animals were then placed with their heads in a soundinsulated box connected to a loudspeaker. After thoracotomy and control of the acid-base balance the first intracardial injection of radioactively labelled microspheres was given and blood samples were taken through free flow from one of the femoral catheters [1]. After this first measurement the animals were exposed to 100 dB SPL white noise for 6 min. In the meantime a second control of the acid-base balance was made, and during the last minute the second blood flow measurement was performed using microspheres labelled with a different radioactive isotope. After the second measurement the animals were put to death by a small dose of KCl intracardially. The cochleas were fixed in phosphate-buffered 2.5% glutaraldehyde and microdissected. The radioactivity of the blood samples, the cochleas and other organs (see below) was counted in a gammaspectrometer and the cochlear blood flow was calculated [1,7]. Two cochleas were excluded: one because there was a middle ear infection, the other because the cochlea was damaged during dissection. The blood flow was also calculated in the cerebrum, the cerebellum, the different parts of the eyes, the masseter muscles, the parotid glands and heart, skin, lungs and kidneys. Only results of particular interest in the present context will be reported here.

The microspheres used were carbonized Latex spheres (3M-Company St Paul, Minn.) with a diameter of 8–10 μm or 15 ± 1 μm and labelled either with ^{141}Ce or ^{85}Sr. The number of smaller spheres injected each time was approximately 15×10^6 and that of the larger ones 8×10^6. The microspheres were suspended in a mixture of saline 0.9% and Macrodex 10% and homogenized by ultrasound treatment just before injection. They were also heated to body temperature. The injected volume varied, depending on sphere size used, between 1.5 and 3 ml.

The noise was generated from a tape recorder (Revox G36 Regensdorf, Zürich, Switzerland) via a power amplifier, Quad 405, to a Philips 9710-M loudspeaker in the box. A specially recorded noise-tape with an equalized signal was used during all the experiments to compensate for the irregularity of the frequency response of the loudspeaker and the box. The tape was prepared by recording the equalized output from a white noise generator (Brüel & Kjaer), after passing a third octave equalizer (Hewlett Packard) and the power amplifier to the loudspeaker. In the box the sound pressure level and the frequency content were measured in the estimated ear position by a calibrated ¼ inch measuring microphone (Brüel & Kjaer), a measuring amplifier 2607 (Brüel & Kjaer) and a third octave real time analyser (Hewlett Packard). By regulating the third octave equalizer for the unlinear frequency response and standing waves in the box it was possible to tape a frequency equalized signal.

Results

The 5 animals which were anesthetized with ketamine-chloride lay motionless with a widening of the eyelids and mydriasis. The effect of sympathectomy was immediately visible: the animals developed miosis and enophthalmos.

The 10 cats which were anesthetized by chloroform-chloralose lay motionless with closed eyes and the effect of sympathectomy was more difficult to evaluate. None of the animals showed visible reactions to the noise. All 15 cats initially had a normal blood pressure between 15kPa and 26kPa. During the injection of the spheres no changes of blood pressure were accepted but some lability was noted during the rest of the sampling minute.

The cochlear blood flow did not show any significant difference between the sympathectomized side and the intact side in the first control measurement. The cochlear blood flow was not appreciably influenced by noise in any of the groups, neither on the sympathectomized side nor at the intact side (fig. 1, 2). 2 animals which had CO_2-retention in spite of the controlled

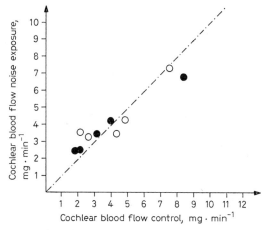

Fig. 1. Cochlear blood flow during noise in correlation to prior control measurement. Unfilled circles indicate sympathectomized side. Filled dots intact side. Ketamine anesthesia.

ventilation are reported separately in table I. This shows a fourfold increase of the cochlear blood flow and no difference between the left and right side.

The cerebral blood flow showed remarkable differences between the two groups, depending on the kind of anesthesia (table II). The mean cerebral blood flow of the ketamine group was $1.32 \text{ mg} \cdot \text{min}^{-1} \cdot \text{mg}^{-1}$ and that of the chloralose group $0.33 \text{ mg} \cdot \text{min}^{-1} \cdot \text{mg}^{-1}$. No differences between the intact and the sympathectomized side in any of the groups were noted. The cerebral blood flow showed a reduction during noise exposure. No effect of noise could be seen on the cerebellar blood flow of the ketamine group but there was a reduction in the chloralose group (table II).

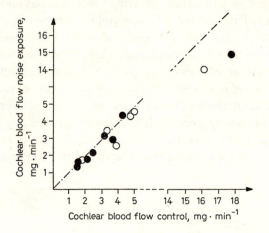

Fig. 2. Cochlear blood flow during noise in correlation to prior control measurement. Unfilled circles indicate sympathectomized side. Filled dots intact side. Chloralose anesthesia.

Table I. The effect of respiratory acidosis on cochlear blood flow

Expt. No.	pH		PCO_2 kPa		Cochlear blood flow $\text{mg} \cdot \text{min}^{-1}$	
	Inj. I	Inj. II	Inj. I	Inj. II	Inj. I	Inj. II
					dx sin	dx sin
5	7.31	7.33	5.81	5.39	16.8/16.8	8.5/ 9.2
10	7.29	7.17	6.99	6.69	17.7/16.1	15.1/14.2

Table II. Blood flow in CNS in relation to anesthetics and noise and sympathectomy (mean and range)

Sympathetic trunk		Ketamine		Chloralose	
		before noise	during noise	before noise	during noise
Cerebrum	intact	1.32 (0.92–2.17)	1.15 (0.66–2.21)+	0.33 (0.17–0.58)	0.26 (0.16–0.42)++
	cut	1.31 (0.94–2.27)	1.28 (0.90–2.35)+	0.34 (0.16–0.59)	0.27 (0.15–0.37)++
Cerebellum	intact	0.58 (0.27–1.16)	0.54 (0.33–0.99) n.s.	0.38 (0.17–0.56)	0.30 (0.20–0.44)+
	cut	0.60 (0.29–1.17)	0.57 (0.35–1.01) n.s.	0.39 (0.18–0.56)	0.30 (0.19–0.43)+

t test for paired observations between the blood flow before and during noise: + = $p < 0.5$; ++ = $p < 0.01$; n.s. = nonsignificant.

Discussion

Based on histological findings [6, 9], direct observations of cochlear blood vessels in living animals [11], clinical results from treatment of noise trauma with low molecular dextran [10] and studies of the effect of noise on PO_2 and PH_2 in endolymph [12, 13], it has been proposed that noise reduces the cochlear blood circulation. In contrast to the above-mentioned investigations, no effect of noise on the cochlear microcirculation could be demonstrated in the present study. One explanation may be divergences in sound pressure levels used and the time of noise exposure. Moreover, the possibility that oxygen tension in the inner ear fluids may be reduced by other mechanisms than by an impaired blood flow should not be overlooked; one possibility of induced reduction in oxygen tension being when the oxygen consumption and demand is raised and there is no compensatory rise in the blood circulation.

Another interpretation, as suggested by *Hawkins* [6], is a redistribution of the cochlear blood by noise resulting in a lowering of blood flow to certain areas of the inner ear. This could not be demonstrated in the present experiments since the microsphere method, as it is today, only reflects the total cochlear blood circulation.

When discussing whether noise induces blood flow reduction in the inner ear, the network of sympathetic nerves accompanying the blood vessels to the inner ear is of utmost interest. It has already been established that sympathetic stimulation causes a reduction of the cochlear blood flow [7, 8]. *Maass* [12] found that sympathectomy diminished the effect of noise on the endolymphatic PO_2 whereas it did not change the PO_2 in animals not exposed to noise. *Maass* interpreted these results as indicating that in stressed situations like noise exposure the sympathetic nervous system has an impeding effect on the inner ear blood flow. In our investigation, sympathectomy did not influence the blood flow. Thus if an adrenergic activity in the cochlear blood vessels was caused by noise it was not of sufficient magnitude to change the blood flow to such an extent that it could be registered by our method. The effect noted by *Maass* [12] on endolymphatic PO_2 in noise-exposed ears might therefore depend on something else than vasoconstriction. *Spoendlin and Lichtensteiger* [16], *Densert* [5] and *Todd et al.* [17] have discussed a direct influence of the adrenergic nerve terminals on the sensory cells. A sympathetically induced inrcease of metabolism in cochlear sensory cells may be hypothetized. In the brain such an effect of adrenergic substances has been reported by *MacKenzie et al.*

[14]. With no increase in blood flow an enhanced metabolism will result in a reduction of available oxygen.

General anesthesia may influence the cerebral blood flow in different ways depending on the type used [3]. As the same might apply to cochlear microcirculation, two types of anesthetics were used in this study: ketamine, a dissociative anesthetic which increases the cerebral blood flow and chloralose which is a generally depressive substance known to reduce the cerebral blood flow. As expected, the two anesthetics affected the cerebral blood circulation in different ways but the cochlear blood flow was largely uninfluenced by these variations in the cerebral blood flow. Noise exposure significantly reduced the cerebral blood flow both in ketamine and in chloralose anesthesia. The mechanism behind this reduction still remains to be elucidated. The effect of noise on the blood flow in CNS, including the cochlear nuclei, will be reported in a forthcoming publication.

Two animals suffered from a carbon dioxide retention (table I), resulting in a fourfold increase of the cochlear blood flow. This increase is in accordance with earlier findings by *Todd et al.* [17] and stresses the importance of controlling the acid-base balance during measurements of the cochlear blood circulation.

Summary

The effect of noise and unilateral transection of the cervical sympathetic trunk on cochlear blood flow was studied in anesthetized cats. The sound pressure level was 100 dB and the exposure time 6 min. Neither noise nor sympathectomy were found to affect the blood flow.

References

1 Alm, A. and Bill, A.: The oxygen supply to the retina. II. Effects of pressure on uveal and retinal blood flow in cats. A study with labelled microspheres including flow determinations in brain and some other tissues. Acta physiol. scand. *84:* 306–319 (1972).

2 Angelborg, C.; Hultcrantz, E., and Ågerup, B.: The cochlear blood flow. Acta otolar. *83:* 92–97 (1977).

3 Bell, G.J.; Hiley, C.R., and Yates, M.S.: The effects of four general anesthetic agents on the regional distribution of cardiac output in the rat. Proc. of the B.P.S., 1977, pp. 126–127.

4 Borg, E.: Tail artery response to sound in unanesthetized rat. Acta physiol. scand. *100:* 129–138 (1977).

5   Densert, O.: Adrenergic innervation in the rabbit cochlea. Acta oto-lar. *78:* 345–356 (1974).

6   Hawkins, J.E., jr.: The role of vasoconstriction in noise-induced hearing loss. Ann. Otol. Rhinol. Lar. *80:* 903–913 (1971).

7   Hultcrantz, E.; Linder, J., and Angelborg, C.: Sympathetic effects on cochlear blood flow at different blood pressure levels. Inserm *68:* 271–278 (1977).

8   Hultcrantz, E. and Angelborg, C.: Cochlear blood circulation studied with microspheres. ORL *40:* 65–76 (1978).

9   Kellerhals, B.: Acustic trauma and cochlear microcirculation. Adv. Oto-rhinolaryng., vol. 18, pp. 91–168 (Karger, Basel 1972).

10 Kellerhals, B.: Pathogenesis of inner ear lesions in acute acoustic trauma. Acta oto-lar. *73:* 249–253 (1972).

11 Lawrence, M.; Gonzales, F., and Hawkins, J.E., jr.: Some physiological factors in noise-induced hearing loss. Am. Ind. Hyg. Ass. J. *28:* 425–430 (1967).

12 Maass, B.: Tierexperimentelle Untersuchungen des sympathischen Einflusses auf die Innenohrfunktion; Habilitationsschrift, Düsseldorf (1977).

13 Maass, B.; Baumgärtl, H., und Lübbers, D.W.: Lokale pO_2- und pH_2-Messungen mit Nadelelektroden zum Studium der Sauerstoffversorgung unter Mikrozirkulation des Innenohres. Archs Otolar. *213:* 439, 214, 109 (1976).

14 MacKenzie, E.T.; McCuloch, J.; O'Keane, M.; Rickard, J.D., and Harper, A.M.: Cerebral circulation and norepeinephrine: relevance of the blood-brain barrier. Am. J. Physiol. *213:* 483–488 (1976).

15 Misrahy, G.; Shinaberger, E.W., and Arnold, J.E.: Changes in cochlear endolymphatic oxygen availability, action potential and microphonics during and following asphysia and exposure to loud sound. J. Acoust. Soc. Am. *30:* 701–704 (1958).

16 Spoendlin, H. and Lichtensteiger, W.: The adrenergic innervation of the labyrinth. Acta oto-lar. *61:* 423–434 (1966).

17 Todd, N.W.; Dennard, J.E.; Clairmont, A.A., and Jackson, R.T.: Sympathetic stimulation and otic blood flow. Ann. Otol. Rhinol. Lar. *83:* 84–91 (1974).

C. Angelborg, MD, Department of Otolaryngology, University Hospital,
S-750 14 Uppsala (Sweden)

Adv. Oto-Rhino-Laryng., vol. 25, pp. 49–53 (Karger, Basel 1979)

A Critical Evaluation of the Glycerol Test in Meniere's Disease

J. Thomsen and S. Vesterhauge

University ENT Department, Rigshospitalet, Copenhagen

Even though *Hallpike and Cairns,* already in 1938, were the first to describe the endolymphatic hydrops histopathologically, the etiologic importance of this observation has not been clearly demonstrated [*Arenberg and Bayer,* 1977]. Most medical therapies have claimed to have some benefit to the patients, but in an extensive review of the world literature concerning Meniere's disease from 1950 to 1975, *Torok* [1977] stated that there is no benefit from any current medical treatment. This statement is also supported by *Schucknecht* [1976] who states: 'I doubt that we could approve of one single drug in the treatment of Meniere's disease'.

In cases of Meniere's disease resistant to medical treatment it has been increasingly common to perform various surgical procedures, labyrinthectomy, vestibular nerve section, ultrasound or cryosurgery, perforation of the footplate, as well as various decompressive procedures of the endolymphatic sac, either actual shunts to the subarachnoidal space or to the mastoid, or mere decompression by removal of bone over the sac. 'Success rate' in most reports varies from about 60 to 80%, regardless of the treatment modality.

In our previous experience with patients with Meniere's disease we have demonstrated in double-blind studies [*Thomsen et al.,* 1976, 1978] that these patients are extremely good placebo responders, and they could be kept, by and large, free of attacks in a rate of 70% on pure placebo medication, even patients who had been selected as previous 'medical failures'. We therefore concluded and postulated that at least to a great extent the claimed effect of the treatment in various reports might be due to a psychological impact on the patients.

From the literature it is apparent that patients suitable for surgery are selected on various criteria, but most reports have in common that the glycerol test, as originally described by *Klockhoff and Lindblom* [1966], is used to pick out patients, who might benefit from surgery.

Since it is our impression that the Meniere patients are very good placebo responders, we therefore wanted to assess, whether psychological factors influenced the outcome of the glycerol test.

Material, Methods and Results

15 patients participated in the trial. 9 were females, 6 males, with an average age of 55 years, range 25–69 years. In order to participate the patients had to fulfil the following criteria: Presence of typical attacks of fluctuating hearing impairment, tinnitus and vertigo, accompanied by nausea, vomiting and pressure in the ears, with at least one attack every 2 weeks, a history no less than 6 months but no longer than 5 years, normal kidney, cardial and thyroid function and no evident allergies. They should be psychically considered normal. The patients had an average duration of disease of 3.4 years. They were given glycerol, 1.5 g/kg, followed by an equal volume of isotonic saline water. The patients were fasting when given the glycerol, and they were tested audiologically before and 3 h after the intake. To the glycerol was added either a taste of orange or blackberries. The patients had the test performed twice on two consecutive mornings. They were told that they were given two different kinds of either fluid-retaining or fluid-depriving medicine, and that we in one situation would expect hearing to deteriorate, and in the other situation hearing to improve. One audiometrist performed all the audiological tests, and was deprived of the information given to the patient. The patients were randomly chosen both for the sequence of information, as well as the two differently tasting solutions.

Figure 1 shows the effect of glycerol with the two instructions. White columns indicate the mean change in three consecutive octave bands with the instruction of expecting improved hearing. It is seen that the majority are indeed obtaining a better hearing. Grey columns indicate the mean change in three consecutive octave bands with the instruction of expecting hearing to deteriorate. Here too, the majority of the patients follows the instruction, rather than getting an improved hearing, which is the case only in 3 patients. Only patients No. 1 and 8 may have a positive glycerol test, ignoring the negative instruction.

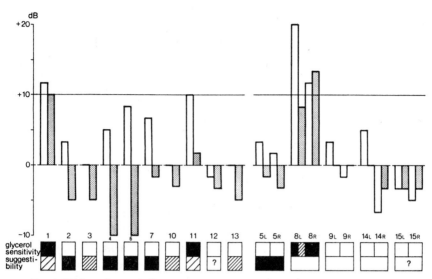

Fig. 1. White columns indicate mean change in three consecutive octave bands with the instruction of expecting improved hearing. Grey columns indicate the corresponding change with the instruction of expecting hearing to deteriorate. Glycerol sensitivity and suggestibility are indicated with black squares.

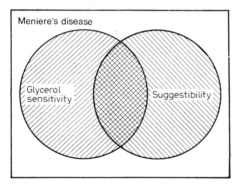

Fig. 2. The total Meniere's sphere with subgroups of glycerol sensitivity and suggestibility.

Discussion

Reviewing the literature we have been unable to find exact information about the diagnostic sensitivity and specificity of the glycerol test. *Klockhoff* [1976] indicates that 'A positive test is indicative of Meniere's disease, whereas a negative test result does not exclude this diagnosis, because the result depends on the phase of the spontaneous course of the disease.' This means that the test processes a high diagnostic specificity and a lower diagnostic sensitivity. We wanted to assess whether psychological factors were responsible or influenced this high diagnostic specificity. In the normal test situation it is virtually impossible to deprive the patient of information as to the purpose of the test. He will definitely inquire why he has to drink such unpleasant fluid, and is invariably told that in case of hearing improvement after the intake he is a candidate for some specific treatment.

Within the framed sphere of Meniere's disease a part of the patients exhibit a glycerol sensitivity, as indicated in figure 2. To this, however, we have to add a circle representing the suggestibility of the patients.

Patients with high suggestibility are probably the same who are good placebo responders. In our trial only 2, maybe 3 patients displayed clear-cut glycerol sensitivity, as seen in figure 1, patients No. 1, 8 and 11 (black squares in the upper row). Patients with clear-cut high suggestibility, those who follow our instructions (indicated with black squares in bottom row) are No. 2, 4, 5, 6, and 7. The more doubtful results are indicated with a hatched square. The 2 cases with question marks experienced severe drowsiness after the glycerol intake, and this can probably explain why they, in both test situations, obtained poorer hearing, due to a reduced alertness.

We believe to have demonstrated that psychological factors do indeed play a very significant role for the outcome of the glycerol test. If this test is continued to be used to select patients for specific treatment, either medical (e.g. diuretic treatment), or surgical (e.g. various decompressive procedures), some alteration in the test procedure is to be recommended. This can either be done in the way of completely depriving the patient of information about the purpose of the test. This is very difficult or most likely impossible. Or the test can be performed in a similar way that we have described. Patients who obtain a better hearing after glycerol intake, in spite of information that we expect the hearing to deteriorate, are true glycerol-sensitive Meniere patients. In these cases for example diuretic treatment seems adequate.

Many authors relate their treatment success rate to the outcome of the glycerol test. Among others, *Arenberg and Spector* [1977] report that of 35 patients operated on, the 8 who had a negative glycerol test did not benefit from surgery. We feel that the selection of patients on the basis of the glycerol test, as it is used today, imposes a risk of selecting exactly those highly suggestible, good placebo responders, who might have benefitted from almost any treatment, or any change in treatment.

Summary

From the literature it is apparent that the glycerol test is being used frequently to evaluate Meniere patients, with regard to the choice of treatment, and in particular to find those who are suitable for surgery with different decompressive procedures. In our previous investigations on such patients we found that they often are extremely good placebo responders and it was natural to evaluate how important such psychological factors would be for the outcome of the glycerol test.

In a group of patients with typical objective and subjective symptoms of Meniere's disease, the glycerol test was applied twice to each patient. In one of the tests, the patient was told that we would expect hearing to improve. In the other test, where the actual amount of glycerol was the same, we had the solution prepared with a different taste, and the patient was informed that we now would expect the hearing to deteriorate. The sequence of the two tests was randomly chosen for each patient. Most frequently the patient would follow our instructions, i.e. obtained a poorer hearing threshold when instructed to, and vice versa. The results are discussed with a special view to the risk of selection of suggestion-sensitive patients by this test.

References

Arenberg, I.K. and Bayer, R.F.: Therapeutic options in Meniere's disease. Archs Otolar. *103:* 589–593 (1977).

Arenberg, I.K. and Spector, G.J.: Endolymphatic sac surgery for conservation of hearing. Archs Otolar. *103:* 268–270 (1977).

Hallpike, C.S. and Cairns, H.: Observations on the pathology of Meniere's syndrome. Proc. R. Soc. Med. *31:* 1317–1336 (1938).

Klockhoff, I.: Diagnosis of Meniere's disease. Archs Oto-Rhino-Laryng. *212:* 309–314 (1976).

Klockhoff, I. and Lindblom, U.: Endolymphatic hydrops revealed by glycerol test. Acta oto-lar. *61:* 459–462 (1966).

Schucknecht, H.F.: In discussion: Medical treatment of Meniere's disease. Archs Oto-Rhino-Laryng. *212:* 384 (1976).

Thomsen, J.; Bech, P.; Geisler, A.; Prytz, S.; Rafaelsen, O.J.; Vendsborg, P., and Zilstorff, K.: Lithium treatment of Meniere's disease. Results of doubleblind crossover trial. Acta oto-lar. *82:* 294 (1976).

Thomsen, J.; Bech, P.; Prytz, S.; Vendsborg, P., and Zilstorff, K.: Meniere's disease: lithium treatment. Demonstration of placebo effect in a doubleblind cross-over trial. Clin. Oto-lar. (in press, 1978).

Torok, N.: Old and new in Meniere's disease. Laryngoscope *87:* 1870–1877 (1977).

Jens Thomsen, MD, University ENT Department, Rigshospitalet, Blegdamsvej 9, DK-2100 Copenhagen (Denmark)

Adv. Oto-Rhino-Laryng., vol. 25, pp. 54–60 (Karger, Basel 1979)

Hearing Improvement in Attacks of Meniere's Disease Treated with Pressure Chamber[1]

Ö. Tjernström, M. Casselbrant, S. Harris and A. Ivarsson

ENT Department, Malmö General Hospital, University of Lund, Malmö

As long as the aetiology of endolymphatic hydrops remains unknown, any treatment has to be symptomatic. At present, we obviously have to accept the fact that we cannot change the natural course of Meniere's disease or arrest the disease. We can only interfere with the attacks.

As to the fluctuant hearing loss, however, there are some interesting clues. By means of a mechanical cochlear model, used in experiments, *Tonndorf* [1957] was able to reproduce the low tone hearing loss by increasing the endolymphatic pressure. His findings indicate that the early fluctuant symptoms of Meniere's disease are mechanical, resulting from a change in the endolymphatic pressure. *McCabe and Wolsk* [1961] have later confirmed these observations in experiments on animals.

Thus, any therapeutic measure that causes a hearing gain, could indirectly be assumed to be due to an effect of a decrease in the endolymphatic pressure.

Exposure of patients with Meniere's disease to underpressure, inducing a relative overpressure in the middle ear, was thought also to reduce the endolymphatic pressure [*Ingelstedt et al.,* 1976; *Densert et al.,* 1975]. This idea emerged from earlier studies in our laboratory. It had been found possible to affect the inner ear function by pressure changes in the middle ear, indirectly by changing the ambient pressure or directly via an eardrum perforation; when increasing the middle ear pressure in normal ears, a vestibular reaction was induced if the overpressure exceeded approximately 60 cm H_2O [*Ingelstedt et al.,* 1974; *Tjernström,* 1977]. It also proved possible

[1] This work was supported by grants from the Swedish Medical Research Council (No. B77-17X-04981-01; B78-17X-04981-02A).

to induce congestion or decongestion of the vascular bed of the middle ear by ambient pressure changes, provided that the middle ear was not in communication with the changing ambient pressure, i.e. the middle ear pressure was kept constant [*Andréasson et al.,* 1976]. A passive opening of the Eustachian tube during ambient pressure decrease and decongestion of the vascular bed could also be observed. In view of these findings we thought it possible to induce variations in volume of the vascular bed in any closed rigid cavity of the body. The question was if similar variations could be produced in the vascular bed of the labyrinth.

Ingelstedt et al. [1976] showed that in some patients it was possible to relieve the symptoms of an acute attack of Meniere's disease very rapidly by exposing them to underpressure. The improvement was confirmed by recordings of spontaneous nystagmus which disappeared in the course of the treatment. This lasted for about 30 min (fig. 1).

One theory may be suggested as an explanation: a reduced pressure outside the body creates a relative overpressure in the middle ear. The magnitude of this overpressure is dependent on the passive opening capacity of the Eustachian tube. As the inner ear is filled with incompressible fluid (fig. 2), the pressure in the inner ear and that in the middle ear will roughly be equal. This pressure transmission from the middle ear to the inner ear might be expected to induce a decongestion of the vascular bed of the inner ear, mainly the venous system.

Evidence for such a pressure transmission has been demonstrated by *Densert et al.* [1978] in animal experiments and *Ivarsson and Pedersen* [1977] have shown that this transmission takes place mainly via the round window. A suddenly increased inner ear pressure due to the above-mentioned mechanism might cause a passive forcing of a temporarily obstructed endolymphatic duct. A prerequisite for such an increase in the inner ear pressure is, however, a poor patency of the cochlear aqueduct to sudden fluid exchange following a sudden pressure change. This theory was discussed in an earlier paper by *Tjernström* [1977].

In a disease known for its spontaneous remissions any therapeutic results have to be appraised sceptically, particularly if the treatment goes on for a long time or if the revaluation takes place several days after the completion of medical or surgical therapy. In the present study we have preferred to find out the immediate effect on low tone hearing loss induced by one single exposure to underpressure. The reason for this is the difficulty in proving the effect of any treatment, even if controls are involved, i.e. excluding a spontaneous remission taking place during the treatment.

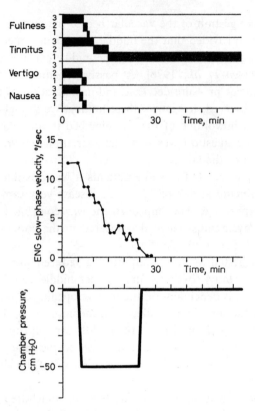

Fig. 1. Schematic presentation of subjective and objective symptoms before, during and after underpressure exposure. Objective symptoms – nystagmus – given as slow-phase velocity. The figures 1, 2 and 3 indicate the severity of subjective symptoms.

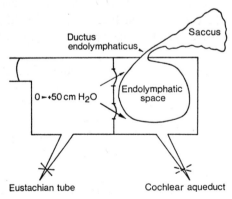

Fig. 2. Schematic presentation of middle and inner ear and the endolymphatic duct and sac. A relative overpressure is induced in the middle ear by ambient pressure reduction, using a pressure chamber. For details see text.

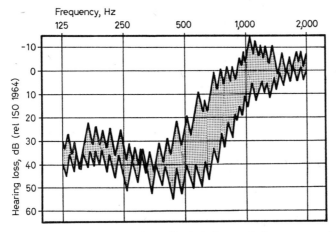

Fig. 3. Bekesy audiograms immediately before and after exposure to underpressure. Dotted area shows the hearing gain.

The criterion for selection was an actual attack with low tone cochlear hearing loss. The treatment was restricted to cases where the actual attack had not lasted for more than 4 weeks.

Results

36 patients fulfilling these criteria were exposed to underpressure on one single occasion for about 30 min. Immediately before and after the treatment, hearing thresholds were registered with Bekesy audiometry. The hearing thresholds recorded by Bekesy audiometry have recently been shown to be much more accurate than those recorded by pure-tone audiometry [*Erlandsson et al.,* 1978]. The middle ear pressure was checked before each hearing test. 17 patients were treated during their first attack and 19 during a recurrent attack.

Hearing improvement was recorded in 15 out of the 36 patients (42%). The criterion for improvement was at least a 10 dB gain for one of the frequencies 250 or 500 Hz. The mean value of improvement was 17 dB. The maximal hearing gain in 1 patient was recorded as 30 dB. Figure 3 demonstrates the hearing gain in 1 patient. Some patients experienced a dramatic relief of all symptoms and none showed additional hearing loss.

In the group of patients who were having their first attack, there was an improvement in 53%, while in the recurrent group the improvement

Table I. Hearing improvement in patients having their 1st attack and in patients having a recurrent attack

	n	Improved	
		n	%
1st attack	17	9	53
Recurrent attack	19	6	32
Total	36	15	42

was 32% (table I). No statistical difference was seen when comparing those who were treated within 1 week, 1–2 weeks or 2–4 weeks of duration of the actual attack.

Among the 15 cases who improved, 3 had a new attack after 4, 12 and 16 months respectively. For the other patients the remission has lasted for more than 1 year in 11 cases and for more than 2 years in 7 cases.

Discussion

The aetiology of permanent hearing loss due to Meniere's disease, like that of endolymphatic hydrops, is unknown. As contributing factors have been discussed metabolic accumulation due to altered endolymphatic flow, chronic venous congestion, diminished arterial flow due to the intralabyrinthine pressure increase and also a mechanical effect on the sensory and neural structures due to distension of the endolymphatic system. There are also animal experiments which suggest that irreversible hair cell damage occurs as early as 6 weeks after the onset of experimentally induced endolymphatic hydrops [Arenberg et al., 1976].

In view of these factors it seems highly important to reduce the endolymphatic volume as soon as possible. Interest has therefore focused on early sac surgery in attempts to save the auditory function in patients with hydrops.

Treatment by underpressure is in line with these ideas and might save the inner ear function in those patients who improve. The treatment is furthermore very easy to perform and does not seem to involve any side effects. It seems unlikely that the demonstrated improvement was a spontaneous remission, particularly not in cases whose actual low tone hearing loss had lasted for 2–4 weeks and who then improved within 30 min in the pressure chamber. The long remission times give further credit to the method.

The aim of this report is to present a method by which it is possible to interfere with an attack of Meniere's disease and to induce immediate improvement of low tone hearing loss in some patients. The improvement is not of the same transient kind as is seen with glycerol and urea intake [*Klockhoff and Lindholm,* 1966; *Angelborg et al.,* 1977]. Some patients have had a period of total remission for more than 2 years. The demonstrated effect might provide additional knowledge as to the cause and pathogenesis of Meniere's disease.

Summary

A method to reduce endolymphatic pressure by exposing patients with Meniere's disease to underpressure has earlier been described. In this work the possible mechanisms are discussed. A material of 36 patients with acute attacks, treated in this way, is now presented. 15 out of these patients experienced a rapid hearing improvement. In 11 cases the remission has lasted for more than 1 year. The method seems to be of great value for those who improved, since at least an early permanent damage to the cochlea can be avoided.

References

Andreasson, L.; Ingelstedt, S.; Ivarsson, A.; Jonson, B., and Tjernström, Ö.: Pressure-dependent variations in volume of mucosal lining of the middle ear. Acta oto-lar. *81:* 442–449 (1976).

Angelborg, C.; Klockhoff, I., and Stahle, J.: Urea and hearing in patients with Meniere's disease. Scand. Audiol. *6:* 143–146 (1977).

Arenberg, I.K.; Murray, J.P.; Rauchbach, E., and Schenk, N.L.: An experimental model for study of endolymphatic hydrops in sharks: implications for the clinician. Laryngoscope *86:* 1426–1434 (1976).

Densert, O.; Carlborg, B., and Stagg, J.: Pressure regulating mechanism in the inner ear (to be published, 1978).

Densert, O.; Ingelstedt, S.; Ivarsson, A., and Pedersen, K.: Immediate restoration of basal sensorineural hearing (Mb Meniere) – using a pressure chamber. Acta oto-lar. *80:* 93–100 (1975).

Erlandsson, B.; Håkansson, H.; Ivarsson, A., and Nilsson, P.: Comparison of the hearing thresholds measured by pure-tone audiometry and by Bekesy sweep audiometry. University of Lund, LUN FD6/(NFFY-3002) LU MEDW/(MERM-3002) (1978).

Ingelstedt, S.; Ivarsson, A., and Tjernström, Ö.: Vertigo due to relative overpressure in the middle ear. Acta oto-lar. 78: 1–14 (1974).

Ingelstedt, S.; Ivarsson, A., and Tjernström, Ö.: Immediate relief of symptoms during acute attacks of Meniere's disease, using a pressure chamber. Acta oto-lar. 82: 368–378 (1976).

Ivarsson, A. and Pedersen, K.: Volume pressure properties of round and oval windows. Acta oto-lar. 84: 38–43 (1977).

Klockhoff, I. and Lindholm, U.: Endolymphatic hydrops revealed by glycering test. Acta oto-lar. 61: 459–462 (1966).

McCabe, B.F. and Wolsk, D.: Experimental inner ear pressure changes. Ann. Otol. Rhinol. Lar. 70: 541–555 (1961).

Tjernström, Ö.: Effects of middle ear pressure on the inner ear. Acta oto-lar. 83: 11–15 (1977).

Tonndorf, J.: Mechanisms of hearing loss in early cases of endolymphatic hydrops. Ann. Otol. Rhinol. Lar. 66: 766–784 (1957).

Ö. Tjernström, MD, ENT Department, Malmö General Hospital,
University of Lund, S-214 01 Malmö (Sweden)

Adv. Oto-Rhino-Laryng., vol. 25, pp. 61–65 (Karger, Basel 1979)

Cat Primary Canal Neurons: Relation of Conduction Velocity to Resting and Dynamic Firing Characteristics

Charles H. Markham, Toshiaki Yagi and Norman E. Simpson

Reed Neurological Research Center, UCLA School of Medicine, Los Angeles, Calif.

The relation between resting and dynamic discharge characteristics in sensory neurons to nerve and receptor morphology has long been of interest. However, it has been difficult to get precise information, particularly in the vestibular system. Two major steps have been made. One is the investigation of *O'Leary et al.* [11] who demonstrated in the isolated labyrinth of the guitarfish a clear relation between primary afferent fiber size and adapting characteristics and sensitivity to angular acceleration. The other work is that of *Goldberg and Fernández* [7] who showed a correlation between regularity of spontaneous firing of primary vestibular afferents in the squirrel monkey with antidromic conduction times.

In the present study of primary horizontal canal afferents, we have compared the functional characteristics, particularly regularity of spontaneous firing and sensitivity to angular acceleration, to the time delay between electrical labyrinthine stimulation and the recording of the evoked action potentials from the afferents in Scarpa's ganglion.

The methods have been outlined in *Yagi et al.* [14]. Briefly, first-order afferents were recorded extracellularly in cats anesthetized with pentobarbital sodium. The functional relationship with the horizontal canal was determined by rotational testing procedures previously described [6]. Unitary recording and amplification were done by conventional means. Conduction times were determined by stimulating between large electrodes placed in the oval and round windows and recording from a glass micropipette placed in the region of Scarpa's ganglion in the superior vestibular nerve. Unitary data, both with regard to the results of stimulation and spontaneous firing, were recorded on film and tape.

The discharge of each unit was noted at rest and then the cat was subjected to a velocity trapezoid in which constant angular acceleration from 2.5 to 19.0°/sec² was followed by a constant velocity of 200°/sec which in turn was followed by deceleration at 4°/sec². Four to six profiles were usually carried out on each unit.

The mean resting rate was 32.4 spikes/sec with a standard deviation of 20.9 and a range from 0 to 84 (n = 177). The regularity of the units was determined by using the coefficient of variation (CV), defined as the standard deviation of the interspike intervals divided by the mean interval. The distribution of CVs enabled the units to be divided into three groups. These were regular firing units with a CV of less than 0.15, intermediate units with a CV between 0.15 and 0.60 and irregular firing units with a CV more than 0.60. Of the 132 units measured, 46% were regular, 31% were intermediate and 23% were irregular. There was a clear correlation between the average resting rate of the regular, intermediate and irregular units with values of 48.7 ± 12.7 (n = 61), 24.5 ± 11.7 (n = 40) and 6.4 ± 6.0 (n = 31) spikes/sec respectively. These groups were from different populations (p < 0.001, using the two-tailed T test).

Sensitivity, the number of spikes/sec/degree of acceleration, defines the unitary activity at a given moment in time for a neuron responding to angular acceleration. Mean sensitivity for the regular, intermediate and irregular units when tested at the same acceleration range was 1.55 ± 0.83 (n = 54), 2.51 ± 1.12 (n = 40) and 2.53 ± 1.82 (n = 28), respectively. The mean sensitivity of the regular firing group was significantly lower compared to the intermediate and irregular groups. However, it should be noted the irregular group contained units with the lowest sensitivity as well as the highest sensitivity of the total population.

The responses of horizontal canal units to prolonged angular acceleration could also be characterized as adapting or nonadapting [2]. In a group of 49 regular units, there were 46 nonadapting neurons while in a group of 21 irregular cells, 15 showed adaptation.

Latencies to electrical stimulation of the ipsilateral labyrinth were measured on 124 units which were functionally characterized as described above. Electrical stimulation intensities of 1.5–2 times threshold resulted in an average response latency of 0.35 ± 0.10 msec with a range of 0.17–0.53 msec. The mean latencies of the regular and irregular groups was 0.4 and 0.2 msec; these are significantly different (p < 0.001) (fig. 1).

Electrical stimulation may excite the nerve via the receptor cells. Indirect evidence supports this in experiments on lateral line organs [3, 12]. On the other hand, in cat single cochlear nerve fibers, the consistently

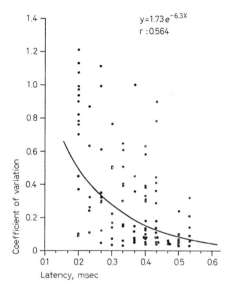

Fig. 1. Coefficient of variation (regularity of spontaneous discharge) as a function of response latency to electrical stimulation in 104 horizontal canal afferent neurons.

shorter latency to electrical stimulation near the round window as compared to click may suggest electrical stimulation acts on the nerve terminals [10]. In the present study the exceedingly short latencies averaging 0.34 msec seem too short for an intervening chemical synapse, and we conclude electrical stimulation acts on the nerve terminals.

The time from electrical stimulation between the oval and round windows until an evoked action potential is picked up from axons of a canal vestibular nerve near Scarpa's ganglion is largely determined by three elements: (1) The time it takes the current to reach the neural site of electrical excitation; this spread of current in a volume conductor is practically instantaneous. (2) The time of spike generation or 'setting-up' time [1, 5, 8]; we use 0.1 msec. (3) The time of conduction in the primary afferent nerve, this being the most significant variable. Taking the range of conduction times in the present experiment and subtracting 0.1 msec for setting-up time, and using a conduction distance of 3.2 mm from the point of stimulation to Scarpa's ganglion, the conduction velocities were calculated to range from 7.4 to 46 m/sec (mean 12.8 m/sec). From this fiber diameters may be calculated to range from 1.2 to 7.6 µm (mean 2.1 µm).

Using the conduction velocities determined above, we can correlate low conduction velocities (and by inference, small diameter axons) with high

Table I. Summary of the data from the present experiment, compared to known morphological characteristics of the crista sensory epithelium

Regularity of spontaneous discharge	Physiological characteristics				Morphological characteristics	
	resting frequency	sensitivity to angular acceleration	adapting response to prolonged acceleration	conduction velocity	fiber size	location in crista
Regular	high	low	nonadapting	slow	thin	slope
Intermediate	medium	medium	mixed	medium	medium	slope summit
Irregular	low	high	adapting	fast	thick	summit

electrical stimulation thresholds, high resting discharge rate, regular discharge, mean low sensitivity to angular acceleration and infrequent adaptation. High conduction velocities (and by inference, large axons) correlate with lower stimulation thresholds, low resting rate, irregular firing, higher sensitivity and frequent adaptation (table I).

Thicker nerve fibers go to the summit of the crista and thinner fibers to the sides of the crista [4, 13]. Since the physiological characteristics in the guitarfish [11] are much the same as in the cat in the present experiment, and since the guitarfish has only Type II receptor cells, it suggests that size and possible ramification of fibers in the crista is more important than the distribution of Type I and Type II receptors as found in mammals [9].

Lastly, thin primary fibers have many branches and innervate many receptors as compared to thick afferents [13]. Recent investigations of Corthoys (personal communication, 1978) suggest that multiplicity of branching may contribute to regularity of firing.

Summary

Spontaneous discharge patterns of first-order canal afferents were analyzed in cats anesthetized with pentobarbital sodium with particular emphasis on the relationship of regularity of resting discharge, sensitivity to angular acceleration and adaptation to the time delay between electrical labyrinthine stimulation and recording from afferents near Scarpa's ganglion. Regular units were found to have a high resting rate, low sensitivity to angular acceleration, were mostly nonadapting during prolonged acceleration and showed relatively long latency to electrical stimulation. Irregular units tended to have a low resting rate, high sensitivity, frequently showed adaptation and had short latencies. Intermediate neurons had mixed characteristics of regular and irregular units.

In medulated nerve fibers, a direct relation exists between conduction velocity and fiber diameter. As latency is due primarily to conduction in the first-order axon, we may speculate that regular neurons have thin fibers which innervate the slope of the crista, irregular neurons have thick fibers which innervate the summit, and intermediate units have medium caliber fibers which innervate both the slope and summit of the crista ampullaris.

References

1   Blair, E.A. and Erlanger, J.: On the process of excitation by brief shocks in axons. Am. J. Physiol. *114:* 309–316 (1935–1936).
2   Blanks, R.H.I.; Estes, M.S., and Markham, C.H.: Physiologic characteristics of vestibular first-order canal neurons in the cat. II. Response to constant angular acceleration. J. Neurophysiol. *38:* 1250–1268 (1975).
3   Dodson, T.; Strelioff, D., and Honrubia, V.: Effects of anoxia on neural activity in the Xenopus laevis lateral line. J. acoust. Soc. Am. *56:* suppl. 11 (1974).
4   Dunn, R.F. and O'Leary, D.P.: Quantitative analysis of nerve fiber distribution within the horizontal ampullary nerve of the guitarfish semicircular canal. Neurosci. Abstr. *II:* 1051 (1976).
5   Erlanger, J. and Gasser, H.S.: Electrical signs of nervous activity; 2nd ed. pp. 82–84 (University of Pennsylivania Press, Philadelphia 1968).
6   Estes, M.S.; Blanks, R.H.I., and Markham, C.H.: Physiologic characteristics of vestibular first-order canal neurons in the cat. I. Response plane determination and restingdischarge characteristics. J. Neurophysiol. *38:* 1232–1249 (1975).
7   Goldberg, J.M. and Fernández, C.: Conduction times and background discharge of vestibular afferents. Brain Res. *122:* 545–550 (1977).
8   Hunt, C.C. and Kuffler, S.W.: Stretch receptor discharges during muscle contraction. J. Physiol., Lond. *113:* 298–315 (1951).
9   Lindeman, H.H.: Studies on the morphology of the sensory regions of the vestibular apparatus. Ergebn. Anat. EntwGesch. *42:* 1–113 (1969).
10 Moxon, E.C.: Neural and mechanical responses to electrical stimulation of the cat's inner ear; thesis MIT (1971).
11 O'Leary, D.P.; Dunn, R.F., and Honrubia, V.: Analysis of afferent response from isolated semicircular canal of the guitarfish using rotational acceleration white-noise inputs. I. Correlation of response dynamics with receptor innervation. J. Neurophysiol. *39:* 631–644 (1976).
12 Sand, O.; Ozawa, S., and Hagiwara, S.: Electrical and mechanical stimulation of hair cells in the mudpuppy. J. comp. Physiol. *102:* 13–26 (1975).
13 Wersäll, J.: Studies on the structure and innervation of the sensory epithelium of the crista ampullares in the guinea pig. A light and electron microscopic investigation. Acta oto-laryng. *126:* suppl., pp. 1–85 (1956).
14 Yagi, T.; Simpson, N.E., and Markham, C.H.: The relationship of conduction velocity to other physiological properties of the cat's horizontal canal neurons. Expl. Brain Res. *30:* 587–600 (1977).

C.H. Markham, MD, Reed Neurological Research Center,
UCLA School of Medicine, Los Angeles, CA 90024 (USA)

Adv. Oto-Rhino-Laryng., vol. 25, pp. 66–73 (Karger, Basel 1979)

Analysis of Nonlinear Afferent Response Properties from the Guitarfish Semicircular Canal

D.P. O'Leary and C. Wall III

Eye and Ear Hospital, Department of Otolaryngology,
University of Pittsburgh School of Medicine, Pittsburgh, Pa.

Introduction

Several decades of experimental research have resulted in new information concerning engineering input-output models of the semicircular canal, but the functional mechanisms of transduction and neural encoding are not understood. Models of receptor dynamics in the form of transfer functions or differential equations have been obtained from linear analysis of experimental response data from stimulation with sinusoidal, constant or pseudo-random rotational acceleration inputs [*Groen et al.,* 1952; *Goldberg and Fernandez,* 1971; *Blanks et al.,* 1975; *O'Leary et al.,* 1974, 1976]. Of particular interest is the diversity of afferent response dynamics observable from the receptor, including adaptation or response decline to a maintained rotational acceleration. A common assumption in these studies is that afferent response dynamics can be considered approximately linear and time invariant. However, it is known that synaptic transmission and subsequent spike train modulation include intrinsic nonlinearities, such as membrane thresholds for impulse generation and afferent impulse rate-limiting phenomena, that could influence obervations of afferent response dynamics.

Our purpose in this study was to determine whether afferent response dynamics were fixed, as would be expected from a linear filter, or could be modified by use of particular combinations of rotational acceleration stimuli. This technique combines a high frequency, or 'dither' signal with a low frequency rotational acceleration input, and this combination acts as a sensitive probe for identifying certain classes of nonlinearities in engineering control systems [*Atherton*, 1975; *Simpson*, 1973]. For example, systems that contain relays or static friction elements in which the output remains at discrete values until an input threshold is exceeded can be linearized for accurate low frequency modulation by application of a high frequency signal. A practical example is the use of small vibrators in jet plane instrument panels to prevent instrument needles from sticking. The presence of a nonlinearity can be determined, and under certain conditions classified, by comparing the response to the dual input with that from the lower frequency (e.g. sinusoidal) input only.

Semicircular canal transduction could include significant effects of nonlinearities from various sources such as viscoelastic phenomena in the cupula and endolymph, synaptic transmission, and afferent membrane thresholds for nerve impulse generation. This report describes our results from the use of a dual input technique which tests for such nonlinearities, and discusses their effects on afferent information processing.

Methods

Isolated labyrinths from the guitarfish *Rhinobatos productus* were prepared for recording afferent responses from the horizontal ampullary nerve using methods described by *O'Leary et al.* [1976]. Extracellular afferent responses from specific regions of the nerve were recorded by the use of forceps electrodes similar to the technique described by *Groen et al.* [1952], which afforded long-term recording stability in the presence of high frequency stimulation. After isolation of a functional afferent unit, a low frequency test signal in the form of either a pseudorandom binary sequence (PRBS) (band limited white noise) or a sinusoidal rotational acceleration stimulus was used in order to determine the linear system dynamics as described by *O'Leary et al.* [1976]. The same afferent unit was then tested using a combined low (0.04–3 Hz) and high frequency (oscillation from 30 to 100 Hz) stimulus, with a servocontrolled rotating table interfaced to a PDP 11 computer. The preparation was aligned so that the horizontal semicircular canal was in the horizontal plane of rotation of the table. It was held rigidly by a simple mechanical clamp bolted directly to the table to eliminate possible spurious harmonics of an elevated superstructure. A sensitive accelerometer (Kistler, Model 305 B, Sundstrand Data Controls, Redmond, Wash.) was used to monitor the stimulus. In one series of experiments, a PRBS rotational acceleration test signal spanning a bandwidth from 0.04 to 4.0 Hz was combined with a 30 Hz 'dither' signal and cross-correlation analysis techniques from nonlinear control engineering were applied to determine nonlinear response interactions to this dual input [*Simpson*, 1973]. The stimulus magnitudes used were 100 and 400°/sec² for the PRBS and dither, respectively. Another dual stimulus used was a combination of a low frequency sinusoid (less than 0.5 Hz) and a high frequency (greater than 30 Hz) oscillatory dither signal. The responses to dual stimuli were then compared with those from the lower frequency stimuli.

Results

Previous studies on this preparation described afferent responses which were grouped into two broad classes. Linear system unit impulse responses (UIRs) from central bundles of the nerve showed rapid decay time constants from an initial maximum amplitude, in contrast with UIRs from extreme bundles of the nerve which showed lower amplitude, delayed maximum responses [*O'Leary et al.,* 1974, 1976]. Typical examples of these two classes are shown in figure 1a and c, respectively, which were obtained in response to the PRBS stimulus alone. As a comparison, figure 1b and d shows the UIRs obtained from the same afferent units in response to the combined PRBS and dither stimulus. In both of the response types, there was a reduction in the major decay time of the response from a maximum toward the baseline. This reduction was typical of the results found in responses from all afferents to the dual input. Another significant effect of the dual input was the undershoot of the baseline shown in the UIR in figure 1b relative to that from the same afferent responding to just the PRBS in figure 1a. Because the amount of baseline undershoot in the UIR indicates the amount of adaptation or response decline that would occur in this afferent unit if a constant acceleration were applied, this result shows that application of the dual input increased the amount of adaptation apparent in this unit. Moreover, it was found in all afferents with this type of UIR that the dual input either caused or enhanced undershoot of the baseline indicating increased adaptation. These results imply that both the dominant time constant and also the degree of adaptation of these units are not fixed parameters of linear system properties of this receptor, but can indeed be modified by a nonlinear interaction of high and low frequency test signal combinations.

In order to focus on detailed effects at specific frequencies, we applied additional dual inputs in the form of combinations of high and low frequency sinusoidal test signals. In engineering applications, dual sinusoidal inputs have been used to determine 'hidden' linear system components by minimizing the effects of nonlinearities to result in 'linearized' responses [*Atherton,* 1975]. We therefore expected the afferent responses to the dual input to be sinusoidal with minimal distortion, but with perhaps changes in peak-to-peak amplitude (or gain) and phase relative to those values observed from just the low frequency input. But we observed the opposite result. The responses to the dual sinusoidal input were found to be more distorted than those obtained from a single input. Figures 2 and 3 summarize a comparison of dual versus single input responses from an afferent with a UIR similar to

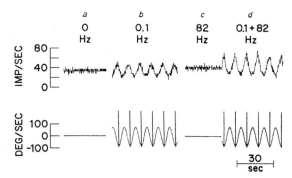

Fig. 2. Nonlinear sinusoidal responses resulting from combined sinusoidal stimuli of 0.1 and 82 Hz. *a* Afferent spontaneous activity. *b* Response of the same unit to a sinusoidal frequency of 0.1 Hz. *c* Response to an oscillatory stimulus of 82 Hz. *d* Response to a combined stimulus of 0.1 and 82 Hz. The lower traces show the 0.1 Hz stimulus velocity, combined with vertical period markers.

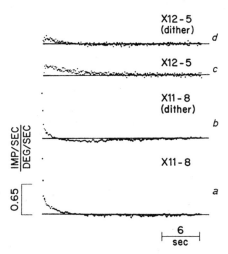

Fig. 1. Effects of a 30 Hz dither oscillation on linear system unit impulse responses (UIRs) obtained by cross-correlation of pseudorandom binary sequence (PRBS) with single afferent responses. *a* Response from unit X11-8 to PRBS stimulus only. *b* Response from unit X11-8 to PRBS combined with the dither signal. A comparison of figure *1b* with *a* shows that a nonlinear interaction of the dither stimulus with the ampullar transduction mechanisms resulted in a more rapid decay from the maximum followed by an undershoot of the baseline. The undershoot reflects adaptation, or response decline, of the afferent unit. *c* Response from unit X12-5 to PRBS stimulus only. *d* Response from unit X12-5 to PRBS combined with the dither signal. A comparison of figure *1d* with *c* shows that the dither resulted in a faster decay time in this class of afferent UIR also. The UIRs shown are representative of two main classes from this preparation [*O'Leary et al.*, 1976].

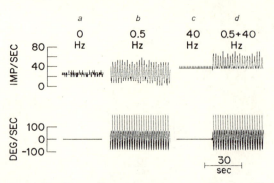

Fig. 3. Nonlinear afferent responses to combined oscillatory stimuli of 0.5 and 40 Hz. The responses are from the same unit as those shown in figure 2. *a* Spontaneous activity. *b* Response to a 0.5 Hz sinusoidal stimulus. *c* Response to a 40 Hz oscillatory signal. *d* Response to a combined stimulus of 0.5 and 40 Hz. The response asymmetry in figure *3d* resembles a half-wave rectifier.

that in figure 1a, but more sharply peaked. The form of equivalent nonlinearity in this afferent response output varied from that resembling a halfwave rectifier (fig. 3d) to an exaggerated positive phase and attenuated negative phase of the output response (fig. 2d). When compared with the responses to just the low frequency test signals (fig. 2b, 3b), these results imply that the effect of a dual input was to greatly enhance a nonlinear effect that was either absent or greatly diminished in the low frequency responses. Moreover, these results were found to be typical in form to those determined from other semicircular canal afferents.

The responses in figure 1–3 were chosen because they illustrate the main effects of the dual input that were observed to a greater or lesser degree in responses from all other afferents in this receptor. In each afferent, the amount of distortion was found to be a variable that was determined by the relative amplitudes and frequencies of each component of the paired input.

Although our observed changes in system, or 'black box' modeling, characteristics are of interest from the perspective of information processing, they result from specific physiological transduction mechanisms that are not well understood. In order to study them, we examined the extracellular afferent response records in detail to determine possible sources of the observed nonlinearities. In figure 4a and b are shown a portion of the spike train response to the dual sinusoidal input (0.5 + 40 Hz) described in figure

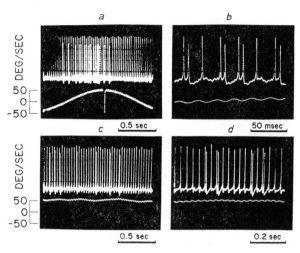

Fig. 4. Detailed representation of nerve impulses resulting from combined stimuli
a Spike train response to one period of the 0.5 + 40 Hz stimulus from figure 3d. The
taller spike responded once per period of the oscillatory dither signal. b Expanded time
sample of the response in figure 4a. Shorter spikes are observed preceded by a taller
spike with a latency of 6–8 msec. c Detail of spike train response to the combined PRBS +
30 Hz stimulus described in Methods. d Time expansion of the response shown in
figure 3c. Both phase locking to the dither signal and also taller-shorter spike doublets
were observed from this combined stimulus also.

3d. Two effects are apparent. First, phase locking occurred in which the cell
fired one spike during each period of the 40 Hz dither signal. Second, during
the excitatory phase of the 0.5 Hz test signal, shorter spikes occurred preceded invariably by a taller spike 5–10 msec earlier (fig. 4b). This time syn-
chrony in doublets implies that the shorter spikes originated from the same
afferent as the taller, and occurred during the cell's relative refractory period.
We therefore conclude from this detailed view of the responses in figure
4a and b that (1) phase locking of taller spikes to the dither signal was
the essential nonlinearity resulting in the diminished response during the
inhibitory phases of the sinusoidal responses shown in figures 2d and 3d,
and (2) that increased excitability led to the taller-shorter spike doublets (i.e.,
more spikes per unit time), which resulted in the enhanced positive phase
sinusoidal responses of figures 2d and 3d. Moreover, the same phase locking
and doublet spike effects occurred during the responses to the combined
PRBS and dither stimuli, as shown by representative samples of these res-

sponses in figure 4c and d. We suggest, therefore, that phase locking and doublet spiking were the cause (at least in part) for the changes in unit impulse responses depicted in figure 1.

Discussion

A major goal in system identification analyses is to infer explicit mechanisms that determine the observable system parameters. Our results suggest the following interpretations at the cellular level. The probabilistic phase locking spike train response resulting from the dither signal can be considered a change in the level of excitability of the hair cell and/or the afferent membrane. The changed membrane excitability resulted in a response asymmetry, as shown by distortion in the sinusoidal responses of figures 2d and 3d, and a similar asymmetry is thought to be the basis for the observed UIR changes at the system parameter level. This process is controlled, at least in part, by the excitability state of the postsynaptic afferent membrane, because our results indicate that excitatory modulation can occur during the relative refractory period, whereas inhibitory modulation is greatly reduced by phase locking to the dither signal.

Although providing a useful probe for identifying receptor nonlinearities in this study, a mechanical dither stimulus is unphysiological with the possible exception of corpuscular flow though capillaries near the hair cells. But our results implying the influence of membrane excitability on the system response parameters suggest an interesting hypothesis concerning a possible role of efferent control in the intact animal. The guitarfish has only Type II hair cells in the crista, in which efferent fibers synapse directly on the hair cells. The state of depolarization of the hair cell membrane would presumably be influenced by the level of activity in the efferents, thus affecting synaptic transmission and excitability in the postsynaptic afferent membrane. On the basis of our above results from combined inputs, we hypothesize that efferent activity resulting in decreased afferent excitability could change the afferent response characteristics to be more sensitive to faster head movements and to have enhanced adaptation analogous to the response changes shown in figure 1b. Conversely, efferent activity resulting in increased afferent excitability would have the opposite effects. In summary, this hypothesis suggests that activity in the efferent system could regulate, or adjust, the form and bandwidth of dynamic afferent response parameters through modification of the state of hair cell and afferent membrane depolarization.

Summary

Nonlinear afferent response properties from the isolated guitarfish semicircular canal were investigated using a nonlinear system identification technique of combined high and low frequency rotational acceleration stimuli. Linear system unit impulse responses obtained from the dual inputs were systematically different relative to those obtained from low frequency stimuli only, implying nonlinear interactions. These results were attributed to neurophysiological mechanisms of phase locking and increased afferent excitability. A hypothesis was proposed in which similar nonlinear interactions could result from efferent activity in intact animals, suggesting that the efferents could act as a regulator of afferent response dynamics.

References

Atherton, D.P.: Nonlinear control engineering (Van Nostrand, New York 1975).

Blanks, H.I.; Estes, M.S., and Markham, C.H.: Physiologic characteristics of vestibular first-order canal neurons in the cat. II. Response to constant angular acceleration. J. Neurophysiol. 38: 1250–1268 (1975).

Goldberg, J.M. and Fernandez, C.: Physiology of peripheral neurons innervating semicircular canals of the squirrel monkey. I. Resting discharge and response to constant angular acceleration. J. Neurophysiol. 34: 635–660 (1971).

Groen, J.J.; Lowenstein, O., and Vendrik, A.J.H.: The mechanical analysis of the responses from the end-organs of the horizontal semicircular canal in the isolated elasmobranch labyrinth. J. Physiol., Lond. 117: 329–346 (1952).

O'Leary, D.P.; Dunn, R.F., and Honrubia, V.: Functional and anatomical correlation of afferent responses from the isolated semicircular canal. Nature, Lond. 251: 225–227 (1974).

O'Leary, D.P.; Dunn, R.F., and Honrubia, V.: Analysis of afferent responses from isolated semicircular canal of the guitarfish using rotational acceleration white noise inputs. I. Correlation of response dynamics with receptor innervation. J. Neurophysiol. 39: 631–644 (1976).

O'Leary, D.P. and Honrubia, V.: Analysis of afferent responses from isolated semicircular canal of the guitarfish using rotational acceleration white noise inputs. II. Estimation of linear system parameters and gain and phase spectra. J. Neurophysiol. 39: 645–659 (1976).

Simpson, R.J.: Use of high frequency signals in identification of certain nonlinear systems. Int. J. Syst. Sci. 4: 121–127 (1973).

D.P. O'Leary, PhD, Eye and Ear Hospital, Department of Otolaryngology, University of Pittsburgh School of Medicine, 4200 Fifth Ave., Pittsburgh, PA 15213 (USA)

Adv. Oto-Rhino-Laryng., vol. 25, pp. 74–81 (Karger, Basel 1979)

Neuronal Responses to Natural Vestibular Stimuli in the Cat's Anterior Suprasylvian Gyrus[1]

L. Deecke, T. Mergner and W. Becker

Department of Neurology and Section of Neurophysiology, University of Ulm, Ulm

Introduction

A cortical vestibular projection in the anterior suprasylvian region of the cat has been described. Electrical shocks applied to the vestibular nerve give rise to short latency field potentials in this region [*Walzl and Mountcastle,* 1949; *Kempinsky,* 1951; *Mickle and Ades,* 1952; *Landgren et al.,* 1967; *Ödkvist,* 1974]. Labyrinthine polarization yields specific neuronal responses in this area [*Kornhuber and da Fonseca,* 1964]. However, natural vestibular stimulation has not been used in previous studies and such stimuli are needed in order to understand the function of this vestibular cortical field. Of particular interest is the input-output relation between the stimulus and the neuronal activity, in order to assess which stimulus parameters (position, velocity, acceleration) are encoded in the cortical neuronal responses. In the present study the response of cortical neurons to horizontal rotation and to tilt was investigated. The responsive cells were located more rostrally than the sulcus in the anterior suprasylvian gyrus (ASSG). An additional point of interest was the interaction between vestibular and somatosensory afferents and their convergence on ASSG neurons.

Methods

Extracellular unit activity was recorded from the ASSG in awake, immobilized and artificially respirated cats using standard methods. Days before the experiment a chronic

---

[1] Supported by the 'Deutsche Forschungsgemeinschaft', SFB 70. Presented at the 6th Extraordinary Meeting of the Bárány Society, London 1977.

head holder and a recording chamber had been cemented on to the skull, and chlorided silver balls had been implanted at the round window of either side. The animals were fixed in a 30° nose down position on a turntable. The following stimuli were used: (1) natural vestibular stimulation: horizontal rotation; dynamic and static tilt around the a.p. axis; tilt of the head with the body stationary.

(2) stimulation of deep somatosensory afferents: tilt of the body with the head stationary; passive deflection of the limbs or vertebral column.

(3) electrical labyrinthine polarization.

Natural stimulation included both sinusoidal and trapezoidal position profiles of various frequencies. Care was taken to avoid (1) visual input by covering the eyes and testing in darkness, (2) acoustic direction cues by plugging the ears and (3) decrease of alertness by monitoring the EEG and using arousal stimuli. Off-line data analysis included average histograms of discharge frequency and their Fourier analysis.

Results and Discussion

Neurons responsive to natural vestibular stimuli were found in a small area midway between the ASSG and the tip of the posterior branch of the ansate sulcus. This study presents preliminary results from 50 neurons all responsive to horizontal rotation. 17 of these were activated by rotation to the ipsilateral side (type I according to *Duensing and Schaefer*, [1958]). 30 cells were activated by contralateral rotation (type II). Type III (activation in either direction) was found in three neurons, whereas type IV (reduction in spike frequency in either direction) has not been observed so far.

The response of a typical vestibular cortical unit to horizontal rotation is given in figure 1. With sinusoidal stimuli the peak of unit activity is almost in phase with ipsilateral peak velocity at 1 Hz (A), whereas with lower stimulus frequencies (B and C) a progressive phase lead can be seen. This is typical for the majority of the cortical type I and type II cells, but a few neurons show a phase lag even at lower stimulus frequencies. The peak increase in discharge frequency above spontaneous firing level (i.e. excitatory gain, if divided by peak input velocity) is larger than the corresponding peak decrease in the other direction. This nonlinearity in unit response becomes particularly evident with the use of trapezoidal stimuli as shown in D. Most of the cortical type I and type II neurons showed this asymmetry. Furthermore, nonperiodic stimulation with rapid acceleration and subsequent deceleration as achieved by the trapezoidal stimulus and as occurring during usual head movements reveals that the rise in unit response is steeper than the decay. As a consequence, the 'phase lead' can be even larger with trapezoidal stimulation than with sinusoidal stimulation

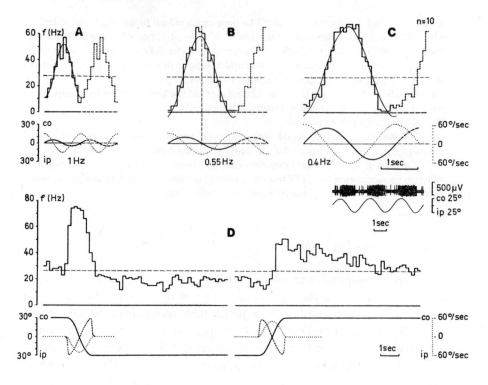

Fig. 1. Vestibular ASSG neuron with type I response to horizontal rotation. The upper curves show the average frequency histograms of 10 periods of rotation. The spontaneous discharge rate is indicated by dashed horizontal lines. The lower curves show the stimulus wave form: angular position (solid line, left calibration marks); angular velocity (dotted lines, right calibration marks), and angular acceleration (dashed lines, in D only). *A–C* Sinusoidal rotation. At 1 Hz stimulus frequency, peak unit activity coincides with peak ipsilateral velocity (A). At lower frequencies (B, C), unit activity slightly leads stimulus velocity. Also shown in histograms A to C is their fundamental wave obtained from Fourier analysis. *D* Trapezoidal stimulation. Note, that (1) modulation in the on- and off-direction is asymmetrical, that (2) the 'phase lead' of the neuronal response is even larger with trapezoidal stimulation as compared to sinusoidal stimuli and that (3) discharge frequency drops rather slowly after stop. Inset below C shows example of original spike data. co = contralateral; ip = ipsilateral.

(cf. D). The long-lasting changes in firing rate after the end of the stimulus are due to the long time constants of the system as observed with ramp velocity stimuli.

21 of the 47 neurons with type I or II response to horizontal stimuli were also responsive to dynamic tilt. The tilt response could be of the same type as the rotational response or of the other type. This convergence of different semicircular canal inputs is shown in the following table which gives the number of neurons and their response types to rotation and tilt.

		Tilt	
		Type I	Type II
Rotation	Type I	3	5
	Type II	9	5

In addition to the convergence of different semicircular canals, convergence of vestibular input with deep somatosensory afferents was observed. These afferents were found to come mostly from neck and limbs. For passive head movement around the tilt axis the response showed the same or the opposite on-direction as compared to the vestibular tilt response.

An example for such convergences is given in figure 2 which shows the same neuron as in figure 1. Whereas the rotational response was of type I, the tilt response was of type II (A). In this particular case there is a clear phase lag in the tilt response as opposed to the phase lead observed in figure 1 with rotation. Sinusoidal tilt of the body alone with the head stationary, as shown in B, which stimulates the neck afferents, apparently gives a similar result with activation in the same direction. However, an isolated body movement in one direction corresponds functionally to a head movement in the other direction (without the labyrinths). Thus, the two inputs are actually antagonistic. When testing the interaction of both inputs, i.e. tilting the head alone with the body stationary (C), there is no complete cancellation of the two inputs. A major reason for this seems to be the difference in phase relation: with neck stimulation alone (B) the peak of unit activity is shifted towards peak position. So far no ASSG vestibular neuron showed consistent responses to *static* tilt of the whole animal or of tilt of body or head alone.

Finally, the same neuron can be activated by passive displacement of the limbs (D) showing activation with retroversion and reduction in spike

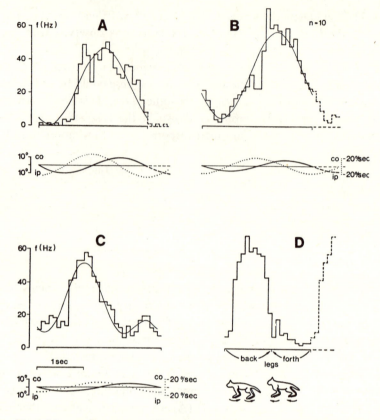

Fig. 2. Neuronal response to tilt and deep somatosensory stimulation. Same neuron as in figure 1 showing type II response to tilt. *A* Tilt of the whole animal. Peak unit activity slightly lags contralateral *velocity*. *B* Tilt of the body with head stationary. Peak unit activity almost in phase with contralateral body *position* corresponding to ipsilateral head rotation without vestibular stimulation. *C* Tilt of the head with body stationary: neck afferents clearly modify the vestibular response. *D* Response to passive anteversion and retroversion of the limbs.

frequency with anteversion. All neurons were tested also with superficial tactile stimuli (touch and hair blowing) but only 1 vestibular cortical neuron showed convergence with hair receptor afferents.

All the cortical neurons responsive to natural vestibular stimuli also responded to polarizing currents applied to the labyrinths. Some more neurons were responsive to polarization but not to the natural vestibular stimuli used. Usually the neuronal response to polarization was related to

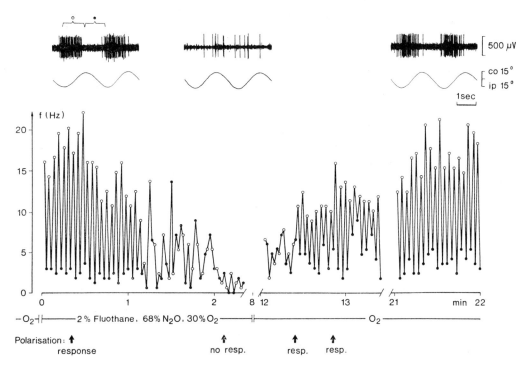

Fig. 3. Effect of anesthesia on the activity of a type II vestibular ASSG neuron. Discharge frequency (ordinate) during contralateral horizontal rotation (activation) and ipsilateral rotation (inhibition) is shown by open and closed circles as indicated in the top insets. Duration of anesthesia is shown on the abscissa. 2 min after onset of the fluothane-N_2O-anesthesia the response to rotation as well as to polarization disappears, and the overall firing frequency decreases. 13 min after the onset of pure O_2 ventilation the vestibular response has recovered.

the polarity of the current and to the side of stimulation (specific vestibular neurons, cf. *Kornhuber and da Fonseca,* [1964]). The response patterns to polarization did not consistently correspond to certain types of rotational (or tilt) responses.

The vestibular neurons of the ASSG area are like other cortical neurons very susceptible to anesthesia. The effect of a general halothane-N_2O-anesthesia on the vestibular neuronal response of a type II ASSG unit is shown in figure 3. Within minutes after the onset of anesthesia the responsiveness of the neuron to both natural vestibular stimulation and labyrinthine polarization is abolished. The recovery of the vestibular responses usually takes considerably longer.

In conclusion, the present investigation has shown that the region of the ASSG represents, indeed, a vestibular projection area in which an integration of different semicircular canal afferents takes place together with deep somatosensory input. The data obtained so far only include responses to *dynamic* vestibular and deep somatosensory stimuli. Concerning a possible functional role of this cortical projection, it seems conceivable that this area elaborates perceptual cues for passive or active movements of head, body and limbs including vestibular and somatosensory information (kinesthesis).

Summary

Neuronal responses to natural vestibular stimulation were recorded in the anterior suprasylvian gyrus (ASSG) of the cat, which in the literature has been proposed as a vestibular cortical projection according to field potentials upon electrical stimulation.

50 neurons were responsive to horizontal rotation. The response generally was directionspecific. Rotation in one direction caused an increase, rotation in the other direction a decrease in spike frequency. On-responses were found for ipsilateral (type I) as well as for contralateral rotation (type II) around the two axes tested. With sinusoidal rotation peak unit activity was usually almost in phase with peak stimulus velocity in the midfrequency range but showed an increasing phase lead at lower stimulus frequencies. Nonlinearities were common in cortical neurons such as a preponderance of the exitatory half wave (particularly evident with trapezoidal stimulation) or a skewness with the rise in unit response being steeper than the decay.

21 of 47 neurons tested were also responsive to dynamic tilt but no consistent responses were observed so far to static tilt. Dynamic tilt of the whole animal (stimulation of labyrinthine receptors) was compared to tilt of the body alone (stimulation of neck afferents) and to tilt of the head alone, resulting in different patterns of interaction of the two inputs in cortical neurons. Convergence of vestibular and proprioceptive input from the limbs was also observed. Responses to natural stimuli were compared to those occurring with electrical labyrinthine polarization. It is concluded that the ASSG cortical area elaborates vestibular information and integrates, in addition to other sensory inputs, in particular deep somatosensory afferents.

References

Duensing, F. und Schaefer, K.P.: Die Aktivität einzelner Neurone im Bereich der Vestibulariskerne bei Horizontalbeschleunigungen unter besonderer Berücksichtigung des vestibulären Nystagmus Arch. Psychiat. NervKrankh. *198:* 225–252 (1958).

Kempinsky, W.H.: Cortical projection of vestibular and facial nerves in cat. J. Neurophysiol. *14:* 203 (1951).

Kornhuber, H.H. and daFonseca, J.S.: Optovestibular integration in the cat's cortex: a study of sensory convergence on cortical neurons; in Bender, The oculomotor system, pp. 239–279 (Hoeber, New York 1964).

Landgren, S.; Silfvenius, H., and Wolsk, D.: Vestibular, cochlear and trigeminal projections to the cortex in the anterior suprasylvian sulcus of the cat. J. Physiol., Lond. *191:* 561–573 (1967).

Mickle, W.A. and Ades, H.W.: A composite sensory projection area in the cerebral cortex of the cat. Am. J. Physiol. *170:* 682–689 (1952).

Ödkvist, L.M.: Vestibular projection to the cerebral cortex. An experimental and comparative study; Linköping University Medical Dissertation No. 24 (1974).

Walzl, E. and Mountcastle, V.: Projection of vestibular nerve to cerebral cortex of the cat. Am. J. Physiol. *159:* 595 (1949).

Prof. L. Deecke, Department of Neurology and Section of Neurophysiology, University of Ulm, Steinhoevelstrasse 9, D-7900 Ulm (FRG)

Adv. Oto-Rhino-Laryng., vol. 25, pp. 82–87 (Karger, Basel 1979)

Effect of Exercise upon Locomotor Balance Modification after Peripheral Vestibular Lesions (Unilateral Utricular Neurotomy) in Squirrel Monkeys[1]

M. Igarashi, J.K. Levy, M. Takahashi, B.R. Alford and J.L. Homick

Department of Otorhinolaryngology and Communicative Sciences, Baylor College of Medicine, and Neurophysiology Laboratory, Medical Sciences Division, NASA-L.B. Johnson Space Center, Houston, Tex.

Introduction

Repeated measurements of locomotor equilibrium function in primates [5] under well-controlled experimental conditions are important because, after partial damage to the body equilibrium system, time-domain functional readjustment occurs due to the existence of multimodal inputs which constantly influence the balance function [6, 8]. In order to modify the labyrinthogenic vertigo and imbalance, *Cooksey* [2] and *Cawthorne* [1] applied physical exercises to the patients after labyrinthine injury, and described that the patients seemed to compensate for their losses better.

This study is to evaluate objectively and quantitatively the impact of enforced kinetic proprioceptive inputs utilizing ataxiametry in the squirrel monkey in which unilateral utricular neurotomy has been placed. Moreover, it could be determined which mode of physical exercise is most effective for balance compensation. Insofar as we did not see any clear effect from exercise application in our previous study of unilateral labyrinthectomy [7], the physical exercise was intensified in this study.

Method

Subjects. Experimental subjects were wild-born squirrel monkeys *(Saimiri sciureus)* of both sexes, approximately 1½–2 years old, and weighing an average of 650 g.

[1] This research was supported by NINCDS grants NS-07237 and NS-10940, and NASA contract NAS-9-14546.

Procedure. The procedure of the squirrel monkey platform runway test was previously described [5, 10]. When the subjects attained the preoperative criterion sequence, animals were randomly assigned to one of three groups. The first group received 1 hour of physical exercise in the squirrel monkey rotating cage (6 rpm). The hour was divided into periods of 10 min of trotting at a constant pace alternating with 5-min rests. The second group was trained to make 60 running shuttles on the squirrel monkey rail (rotating at 200 rpm speed) as a daily exercise. This latter task, a more impulsive and intensive maximum agility problem, contrasts with the continuous and constant, yet less impulsive, trotting given by the rotating cage. The third control group received no physical exercise. Preoperative exercise (or nonexercise) period extended for 3 weeks. Postassignment platform testing continued at 3 times per week.

The surgical procedure of the unilateral utricular nerve resection was similar to the one described in our previous report [4]. Following the operation, all monkeys were tested daily; and thereafter, those receiving exercise were again exposed to daily exercises as scheduled until they reattained preoperative criteria. When the subject regained preoperative criterion, intracardiac fixative perfusion was performed. Temporal bones were processed according to the standard temporal bone preparation procedure.

Results

The overall average of utricular nerve cut was 88 % and the intergroup difference was very minimal. There were some blood cells around the surgical site in one or two ears in each group. One ear had a minute interruption of the membranous labyrinth adjacent to the area of utricular neurotomy, but in all other ears, the membranous labyrinth was intact and utricular neurotomy was done without opening the utricular space. The crista ampullaris superior, crista ampullaris lateralis, crista ampullaris posterior and macula sacculi, and the membranous labyrinth adjacent to those structures showed no remarkable change. There was no collapsed membranous labyrinth. One animal (which belonged to the control group) showed diffuse labyrinthine reaction; therefore, was excluded from the data analysis.

When the average total deviation counts were compared among three groups between postoperative day 1 through day 10, the reduction in both exercise groups was slightly faster than that in the control nonexercise group. This finding may demonstrate some effectiveness of physical exercise toward the reduction of degree of locomotor imbalance in early postoperative stage. The difference in reduction rate between two exercise groups was not remarkable, however.

The mean postoperative calendar days for reattainment of preoperative criteria (a sequence of good performances) were 17.3 days for the rotating cage exercise group, 19.4 days for the rail-traversing exercise group, and

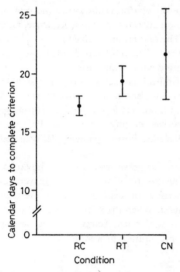

Fig. 1. Comparison of the number of calendar days to reattain preoperative per-formance criterion sequence between rotating cage exercise group (RC), rail-traversing exercise group (RT), and control nonexercise group (CN). Vertical bars represent the SEM.

23.3 days for the nonexercise control group (fig. 1). The largest standard error of the mean was found in the control nonexercise group. When the number of those days were comparatively evaluated by analysis of variance, the three groups' samples did not significantly differ ($p < 0.25$). On the other hand, an analysis of first days of good performance level reacquisition yielded a borderline significant difference ($0.05 < p < 0.10$) overall. When groups were compared by Duncan's multiple range test, the rotating-cage exercise group differed from the control group ($p < 0.05$). The trends between groups with regard to differences in time to functional compensation seemed greater than chance, and suggest the possible presence of an exercise effect. Further intensification of the physical exercise is needed in order to identify clearer differences among the groups.

Postoperatively, a slight increase (about 28 %) of the platform travers-ing time was noted. However, it was equally distributed among three groups, and showed a nonsignificant difference ($F < 1$) between groups. When a correlation was studied (across all subjects) between running time and the number of days to reattain preoperative performance level, a low value was determined ($r = -0.22$). Therefore, as far as the intergroup comparison is concerned, this variable was discounted.

Discussion

It has been reported that the joint receptors play a prominent role in supplying postural information to the vestibular nuclei [11]. Many neurons in the vestibular nuclei are known to be influenced (mainly excitatory) by stimulation of the spinal cord [12]. There is no doubt that interaction of propriceptive and vestibular impulses within the vestibular nuclei complex is important for the maintenance of locomotion and posture. In the Deiters' nucleus, the deiterospinal tract that originates from the rostroventral portion receives primary vestibular afferents, including fibers from the macula utriculi. The essential function of this relay is a reflex maintenance of head position. The deiterospinal tract that originates from the dorsal portion of this nucleus does not receive primary vestibular afferents, instead receives excitatory spinal inputs, which come from lumbosacral spinal cord, and hindlimb muscles. Thus, the hindleg exercise should contribute through this pathway. Also, this particular spinodeitero-spinal reflex pathway receives inhibitory control from the vestibulocerebellum.

Regarding the animal's locomotor behavior, *Schaefer and Meyer* [13] stated that afferent inputs from the hand seem to accelerate the compensation after unilateral vestibular lesions in monkeys. Their observation is in agreement with the results obtained in this experiment.

In our previous experiment, examining the exercise effect upon locomotor dysequilibrium after unilateral labyrinthectomy, we could not detect a clear difference in the postoperative compensation between exercise and nonexercise groups. In the present investigation, many matters were different. First, in our previous study the locomotor balance was measured by the squirrel monkey rail test, whereas in this study we used the squirrel monkey platform runway test which is a deviation measurement of the animal's trot. The previous study was to evaluate the condition after unilateral labyrinthectomy whereas in this experimental series, we investigated the status after unilateral utricular nerve section, which was a smaller lesion. Thus, in this study, animals were less physically (and psychologically) involved postoperatively. Furthermore, in the previous study, the exercise was applied only postoperatively, whereas in this study, we added a preoperative 3-week period. Therefore, in the present study, locomotor balance measurement was done in a more natural form, the vestibular lesion was less stressful to the animal, and, most importantly, a more extended time period of exercise was given, pre- and postoperatively. We further plan to extend the duration (days) of physical exercise so that we can see a clearer effect in the subsequent experiments.

The effects of inhibiting proprioceptive input in experimental animals, by restraint, was reported by *Lacour et al.* [9]. They found that, in alert baboons after the unilateral vestibular neurotomy, postoperative disorders in posture and locomotion are reduced much later when animals are submitted to a motor restriction. *Haines'* study [3] on the effect of 2 weeks of bed rest (in man) showed significant body balance decrements. Those two studies reversely confirm the contribution from proprioceptive inputs toward the postoperative balance readjustment.

Summary

In this study, we placed unilateral utricular nerve section and measured the loco-motor equilibrium function (deviation counts of the animal's trotting gait) by the squirrel monkey platform runway test. We applied physical exercise, both preoperatively (3 weeks) and postoperatively. 21 young adult squirrel monkeys were randomly assigned to three groups (7 each): rotating cage exercise (continuous trotting in the motor-driven rotating cage) group, rail-traversing exercise (60 running shuttles on the rotating rail) group, and control nonexercise group. After the statistical analyses on data it was found that the physical exercise showed some effect; however, the type, daily amount, and number of days applied must be quite substantial.

References

1   Cawthorne, T.: Vestibular injuries. Proc. R. Soc. Med. *39:* 270–273 (1946).
2   Cooksey, F.S.: Rehabilitation in vestibular injuries. Proc. R. Soc. Med. *39:* 273–275 (1946).
3   Haines, R.F.: Effect of bed rest and exercise on body balance. J. appl. Physiol. *36:* 323–327 (1974).
4   Igarashi, M.; Miyata, H., and Alford, B.R.: Utricular ablation and dysequilibrium in squirrel monkeys. Acta oto-lar. *74:* 66–72 (1972).
5   Igarashi, M.: Squirrel monkey platform runway test. A preliminary report. Acta oto-lar. *77:* 284–288 (1974).
6   Igarashi, M.; Kato, Y.; Alford, B.R., and Levy, J.K.: Macular deafferentation and locomotor equilibrium control in squirrel monkeys; in Morimoto, Proc. Barany Society 1975, pp. 36–41 (Barany Society, 1975).
7   Igarashi, M.; Alford, B.R.; Kato, Y., and Levy, J.K.: Effect of physical exercise upon nystagmus and locomotor dysequilibrium after labyrinthectomy in experimental primates. Acta oto-lar. *79:* 214–220 (1975)
8   Igarashi, M. and Alford, B.R.: Animal behavioral studies of equilibrium; in Tower, The nervous system, vol. 3: Human communication and its disorders, pp. 125–135 (Raven Press, New York 1975).

9 Lacour, M.; Roll, J.P., and Appaix, M.: Modifications and development of spinal reflexes in the alert baboon *(Papio papio)* following an unilateral vestibular neurotomy. Brain Res. *113:* 255–269 (1976).

10 Levy, J.K. and Igarashi, M.: Baseline running on a straight platform by squirrel monkeys. Percept. Mot. Skills *45:* 295–300 (1977).

11 Pompeiano, O.: Spinovestibular relations. Anatomical and physiological aspects; in Brodal and Pompeiano, Basic aspects of central vestibular mechanisms, pp. 263–296 (Elsevier, Amsterdam, 1972).

12 Precht, W.: The physiology of the vestibular nuclei; in Kornhuber, Handbook of sensory physiology, vol. VI/1: Vestibular system, part 1, pp. 353–412 (Springer, Berlin 1974).

13 Schaefer, K.P. and Meyer, D.L.: Compensation of vestibular lesions; in Kornhuber, Handbook of sensory physiology, vol. VI/2: Vestibular system, part 2, pp. 463–490 (Springer, Berlin 1974).

M. Igarashi, MD, Department of Otorhinolaryngology and Communicative Sciences, Baylor College of Medicine, Houston, TX 77030 (USA)

Adv. Oto-Rhino-Laryng., vol. 25, pp. 88–92 (Karger, Basel 1979)

Height Vertigo and Human Posture[1]

T. Brandt, W. Bles, F. Arnold and T.S. Kapteyn

Neurological Clinic with Clinical Neurophysiology, Krupp Hospital, Essen and ENT Department, Free University Hospital, Amsterdam

Introduction

Hitherto height vertigo had been attributed mainly to psychopathological processes like neurotic acrophobia [*Purkinje,* 1820; *Kobrak,* 1924; *Takeya et al.,* 1979]. However, height vertigo is a visually induced syndrome of discomfort, commonly experienced on high buildings or in the mountains. It is associated with a subjective instability of free stance and locomotion coupled with a fear of falling and vegetative symptoms.

We believe that height vertigo does not simply represent an unpleasant visual epiphenomenon. Rather, it is a meaningful warning signal to the body (in a teleological sense) for withdrawal from stimulus situations which cannot be adequately perceived in terms of space constancy. And it is space constancy as well as the continuous evaluation of the reafferent sensory consequences of self-generated body movements which provide postural balance. A theory is presented that supports a simple geometrical explanation for physiological height vertigo being a distance vertigo, separate and apart from purely cognitive or psychological factors. It is suggested, that it is a visual destabilization of postural balance, which induces height vertigo, when the distance between the observer and visible stationary contrasts becomes critically large [*Brandt,* 1976; *Brandt et al.,* 1978; *Bles et al.,* 1978].

Height vertigo, a Distance Vertigo Through Postural Imbalance

There are three main loops which control posture, namely (1) the vestibular, (2) the somatosensory and (3) the visual loop. Vision plays a

[1] Supported by 'Deutsche Forschungsgemeinschaft', Br 639/1 'Bewegungskrankheit'.

powerful role within the multiloop control of postural stabilization. It attenuates self-generated sway by 50–100% [*Edwards*, 1946; *Travis*, 1945]. Foreaft body sway can be compared to the motion of an inverted pendulum as a first approximation [*Nashner*, 1970]. Lateral sway, however, is horizontal over several centimeters (parallel shift) because of the joint mechanics [*Kapteyn*, 1973]. In order to maintain postural stability in the upright position afferent visual signals must be generated as an input for compensation of foreaft as well as lateral sway. A lateral sway causes a retinal shift of the visible surround on the retina.

A geometrical analysis indicates that to be visually detected body sway must increase with increasing distance between the eyes and the nearest stationary contrasts (fig. 1). Angular displacement α on the retina is smaller the greater the distance y to the object becomes. Since normal lateral head sway is about 2 cm in amplitude [*Kapteyn*, 1973] the question arises at which particular eye-object distance this sway amplitude cannot be visually detected. If it is assumed that an angular displacement of the visual scene of 20 min of arc is necessary for detection by the paracentral and peripheral parts of the retina [*Leibowitz*, 1955], a lateral head sway of 2 cm is subthreshold at a distance of about 3 m. This leads to a perceptual conflict: the vestibular and somatosensory receptors are sensing a body shift which the visual system cannot detect. The misleading visual signal is that of no change in position relative to the surround. The conflict might be resolved by increasing postural sway and thereby reactivating visual control, but with a decrease in accuracy of postural balance. As a consequence postural instability would occur which secondarily induces subjective height vertigo as a reasonable reaction to high altitudes or great distances. For a simple loop control a relationship between distance and sway amplitude could be expected (tan $\alpha = \frac{x}{y}$), with the gain dependent on the retinal movement detection threshold. However, with the legs close together at free stance, one will fall over at a sway of the head more than 10 cm. Thus, at an eye-object distance of 15–20 m a 'maximal body sway' would produce retinal angular deviations α less than 20 min of arc according to the trigonometrical model. Since we are dealing with a multiloop control of postural balance, it can be assumed that with increasing sway amplitudes the particular sensory weight of the somatosensory and vestibular afferences becomes greater. This will also increase their contribution to postural stabilization. Experiments with the swaying room demonstrated that optokinetically induced head sway saturates at amplitudes greater than 2 cm indicative of a proprioceptive interference [*Bles et al.*, 1977].

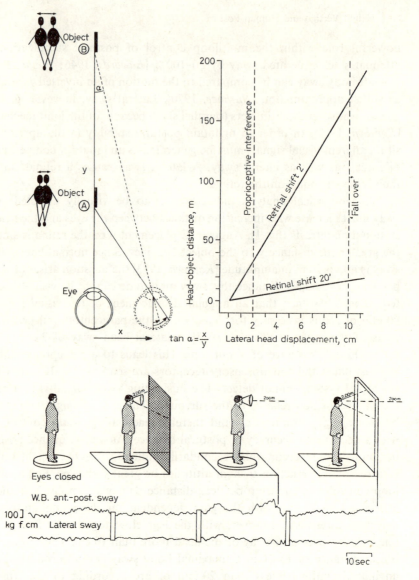

Fig. 1. Geometrical analysis showing that by increasing the distance between eyes and stationary surroundings body sway must also increase in order to be visually detected and to be used for postural stabilization. Lateral head displacement as a function of eye-object distance for assumed retinal displacement thresholds of either 20 or 2 min of arc. Foreaft and lateral body sway (original traces) at eyes closed, eyes open in front of a wall, eyes open on a high building with and without additional stationary contours in the peripheral visual field. Sway amplitudes increase under height vertigo conditions especially in the low frequency range. Simultaneous nearby stationary contrasts in the seen periphery stabilize 'height vertigo sway'.

The geometrical model has been developed for afferent motion perception during lateral horizontal body sway. It must also be valid for efferent motion perception because the thresholds of movement detection are not lower with eye pursuit and 'stabilized retinal images'. It also holds for foreaft sway in which the retinal image of a seen object varies in size respectively.

Psychophysical and posturographic experiments were performed under natural conditions on high buildings to support the theoretical explanation. Surprisingly enough, most of the predictions based on the model were confirmed by the experimental data although we expected additional cognitive factors (independent from the retinal deficiency) to interfere with the basic physiological mechanism in a nonpredictable manner.

Consistent with the geometrical model the results were: (1) the occurrence of height vertigo is clearly related to body position being the strongest with free upright stance when keeping balance is the most difficult; (2) height vertigo can be induced either by downward or upward gaze; it is the distance rather than the visual direction that is critical; (3) its strength increases with increasing distance and saturates at 15–20 m. Thus, height vertigo is already maximal at an altitude of about 20 m; (4) the measurable (foreaft and lateral) body sway increases significantly with increasing eye-object distance as reported earlier by *Lee and Lishman* [1975]. Under height vertigo conditions it is especially affected in the low frequency range <0.1 Hz (fig. 1); (5) nearby stationary contrasts in the periphery of the visual field improve the sway according to the earlier finding that the retinal periphery dominates dynamic spatial orientation and postural balance [*Brandt et al.*, 1973; *Dichgans and Brandt*, 1978]; (6) head tilt (by which the otoliths are brought out of their optimal working range) or additional disturbances of the somatosensors (standing on a soft foam rubber platform) enhance the 'height vertigo sway' because the false visual signal seems to receive a greater sensorial weight.

These results also provide some practical possibilities to alleviate perceptual and postural problems in persons susceptible to height vertigo. Physiological height vertigo must be differentiated from the neurotic acrophobia or height anxiety in which the altitude acts only as the inducing stimulus situation for a pathological phobic reaction as the wide open space in agoraphobia or the fear of confined spaces in claustrophobia.

Summary

A theory is presented supporting a geometrical explanation for physiological height vertigo being a distance vertigo through visual destabilization of postural balance when the distance between the eyes and visible stationary contrasts becomes critically large. Physiological and posturographic data obtained under natural height vertigo conditions are consistent with this hypothesis.

References

Bles, W.; Kapteyn, T.S., and De Wit, G.: Effects of visual vestibular interaction on human posture. Adv. Oto-Rhino-Laryng., vol. 22, pp. 111–118 (Karger, Basel 1977).

Bles, W.; Brandt, T.; Kapteyn, T.S. et Arnold, F.: Le vertige de hauteur, un vertige de distance par une déstabilisation visuelle? Agressologie *19:* B, 63–64 (1978).

Brandt, T.: Optisch-vestibuläre Bewegungskrankheit, Höhenschwindel und klinische Schwindelformen. Fortschr. Med. *94:* 1177–1182 (1976).

Brandt, T.; Arnold, F.; Bles, W., and Kapteyn, T.S.: Height vertigo, a distance vertigo through visual destabilization of free stance; in Kommerell, Disorders of ocular motility. Neurophysiological and clinical aspects, pp. 291–298 (Bergmann, München 1978).

Brandt, T.; Dichgans, J., and Koenig, E.: Differential effects of central versus peripheral vision on egocentric and exocentric motion perception. Expl. Brain Res. *16:* 476–491 (1973).

Dichgans, J. and Brandt, T.: Visual-vestibular interaction: effects on self-motion derception and postural control; in Held, Leibowitz and Teuber, Handbook of sensory physiology, vol. VIII Perception, pp. 753–804 (Springer, Berlin 1978).

Edwards, A.S.: Body sway and vision. J. exp. Psychol. *36:* 526–535 (1946).

Kapteyn, T.S.: Het staan van de Mens; thesis Amsterdam (1973).

Kobrak, F.: Über den Bergschwindel und andere praktisch wichtige Schwindelphänomene. Mschr. Ohrenheilk. Lar.-Rhinol. *58:* 126–134 (1924).

Lee, D.N. and Lishman, J.R.: Visual proprioceptive control of stance. J. Hum. Movem. Stud. *1:* 87–95 (1975).

Leibowitz, H.W.: The relation between the rate threshold for the perception of movement and luminance for various durations of exposure. J. exp. Psychol. *49:* 209–214 (1955).

Nashner, L.M.: Sensory feedback in human posture control. MVT 70-3, Cambridge, Mass.: Man Vehicle Lab MIT (1970).

Purkinje, J.E.: Beiträge zur näheren Kenntnis des Schwindels aus heautognostischen Daten. Med. Jb. (Österreich) *6:* 79–125 (1820).

Takeya, T.; Yasuda, K.; Watanabe, S.; Ohno, Y., and Ushio, N.: A statokinesimetric study of acrophobia. Effects of psychological and visual factors. Agressologie (in press, 1979).

Travis, R.C.: An experimental analysis of dynamic and static equilibrium. J. exp. Psychol. *35:* 216–234 (1945).

Th. Brandt, MD, Neurological Clinic with Clinical Neurophysiology,
Krupp Hospital, D-4300 Essen (FRG)

Adv. Oto-Rhino-Laryng., vol. 25, pp. 93–99 (Karger, Basel 1979)

Vertigo and Dizziness Reflecting Functional Disorders

Alf Nilsson, Nils-Gunnar Henriksson, Per-Åke Magnusson and Lars-Erik Afzelius

Department of Otorhinolaryngology, University Hospital of Lund, Lund

Introduction

Vertigo and dizziness may be attributable to somatic disorders but may also be functionally caused [*Sloane*, 1967; *Afzelius*, 1975; *Henriksson and Afzelius*, 1975; *Magnusson et al.*, 1977]. In clinical work of ours it is often difficult to clarify the 'cause-and-effect' relations between dizziness and functional disturbances. This is due to the fact that in some patients an outburts of somatically caused vertigo may accentuate various functional symptoms. Part I of the present paper is a summary of our previous papers [*Afzelius*, 1975; *Afzelius et al.*, 1978] where efforts to differentiate between patients whose nervous symptoms precede vertigo and those whose vertigo precede nervous symptoms are described. The approach there is based upon an analysis of the nervous symptoms and of the various characteristics of dizziness and vertigo. Part II presents a psychological approach to the study of functional or psychogenic vertigo. Thus, the present paper concerns the problem of dizziness in relation to functional disturbances. The aims of the investigation are to seek answers to the following questions:

(1) How frequently is functional vertigo or dizziness encountered in otologic practice?

(2) Are vertigo and dizziness of a different character in patients with many functional symptoms than in patients without such symptoms?

(3) Can a psychological test-battery reveal differences between vertiginous patients with functionally caused symptoms and normal controls?

(4) Can a psychological test-battery reveal differences between psychogenic vertigo patients who were nervous before, and those nervous only after the onset of vertigo or dizziness?

Material and Methods

The material consisted of 338 patients consulting our clinic in Lund for dizziness. The patients were administered a questionnaire consisting of 95 questions, each question involving up to five alternative answers. The questions aimed at assessing the social and medical background of the patients as well as at analyzing their vertigo, dizziness and related symptoms. The patients were asked to state whether or not they possessed each of ten 'functional' symptoms: depression, irritation, nervousness, previous ulcer, anxiety and panic, lump in the throat, vertigo when lining up, oppression on the chest, palpitations of the heart, oppression on the top of the head.

They were also presented with descriptions of a number of alternative characterizations of their sensations of vertigo and dizziness. Only three of these alternatives – spinning sensation outside the head, turning sensation inside the head and a swaying sensation – showed positive correlations with other findings or symptoms [Afzelius, 1975; Henriksson et al., 1976].

One group of 109 patients with no functional symptoms, another group of 109 patients with three or more functional symptoms, which all appear *before* the onset of vertigo and dizziness, and a third group of 29 patients with two or more functional symptoms all appearing *after* the onset of vertigo or dizziness, were selected from the material. Thus, these latter patients did not show any functional symptoms before the onset of vertiginous symptoms or dizziness [Afzelius et al., 1978].

Results

Men and women are equally common in the group without functional symptoms, whereas women are more frequent in patients with early functional symptoms, and even more so in patients with late.

How the three main characteristics of vertigo and dizziness – a spinning sensation outside the head, a turning sensation inside the head and a swaying sensation – are distributed among the two groups, those with and those without functional symptoms, is shown in figure 1.

In patients without symptoms of nervousness, vertigo was most frequently perceived as a spinning sensation outside the head. In patients with functional symptoms, a turning sensation inside the head and a swaying sensation are more common than that of a spinning outside the head, this difference being more pronounced in subjects whose symptoms appear after than in those in which they appear before the onset of vertigo.

This difference with respect to sensations of vertigo or dizziness in patients with early and with late functional symptoms could be taken to reflect two different types of functional disorders. To examine this possibility a conventional otoneurologic check-up and a psychological test approach were employed.

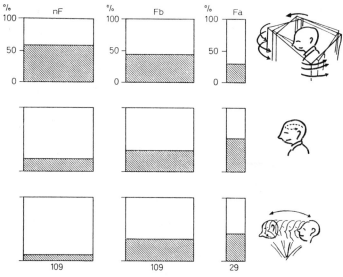

Fig. 1. Characteristics of vertigo and dizziness in patients with and without functional symptoms before and after onset of vertigo and dizziness.

The point of departure for the psychological test approach was the observation that feelings of dizziness contain properties similar to those of feeling of anxiety. Both are commonly reported as diffuse, nonspecific experiences without attachment to a clear-cut and real point of reference. This similarity also constitutes the basis for our efforts to understand psychogenic vertigo as a neurotic symptom.

Figure 2 presents a scheme in which psychogenic vertigo is systematically described in relation to different kinds of (a) *anxiety reactions* [cf. *Nilsson, 1977*], (b) *defensive measures* directed against anxiety. As regards (c) *neurotic symptoms,* psychogenic vertigo is considered in relation to the well-known neuroses of (a) conversion hysteria, (b) anxiety hysteria (phobia), and (c) obsessional neurosis. The scheme also has the aim of presenting those key concepts which will be utilized for describing psychogenic vertigo in that which follows.

Descriptive Instruments

Two experimental techniques and the questionnaire already referred to are employed here [cf. *Magnusson et al., 1977*]:

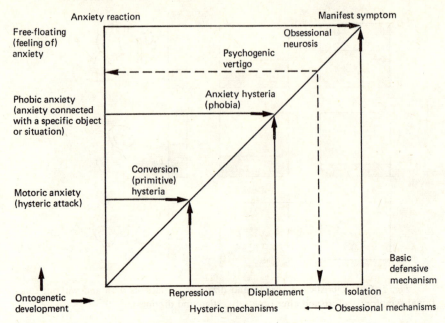

Fig. 2. A schematic description of psychogenic vertigo in relation to conversion hysteria, anxiety hysteria, and obsessional neurosis.

(1) *The Meta-Contrast Technique* (MCT) [*Smith et al., 1970*] involves tachistoscopic presentation of pairs of stimuli in order to study the development of one percept (A) within the framework of another stabilized percept (B). The A-stimulus is an ugly face implying a threat directed against B, a boy sitting at a table with a small window in the upper right corner. First the B-stimulus is presented at gradually prolonged exposure times (initial values = 10 msec) until it is correctly reported. The exposure time is then reduced to a standard level, five exposures at this level then constituting a control series. In the main series, directly after the control series, the A-stimulus is exposed immediately before the B-stimulus at the place of the window in B. A is gradually prolonged (initial value = 10 msec), while the exposure time of B is kept constant, until A+B have been correctly reported in three consecutive trials.

Scoring dimensions are as follows: free-floating *anxiety:* scored when subjects report dark formations; *defence mechanisms:* (a) *repression* (conversion hysteria): the threat (A) is seen as a flowerpot for example; (b) *displacement* (anxiety hysteria): the threat is seen, e.g., as a bare tree; (c) *isolation* (obsessional neurosis): e.g., a barrier between the threat and the boy is reported.

(2) *Spiral after-effect experiment* (SAE) [*Andersson et al.,* 1970] involves measurements of the duration of apparent sensation after the subject has been exposed to a rotating, so-called Archimedes spiral for 45 sec. The experiment comprises ten repeated trials. The development of the durations over trials have in previous studies [*Andersson et al.,* 1972] shown patterns which seem to reflect different types of personality styles. The only relevant pattern in the present study is that which implies a short initial duration followed by successively decreasing durations over the ten trials. This pattern is associated with an hysteric personality style.

(3) *Questionnaire.* Relevant for the present study are the items dealing with: (a) functional symptoms (anxiety), (b) vertigo or dizziness sensation (turning sensation inside the head, spinning sensation outside the head, swaying sensation), (c) characteristics of the first dizziness sensation (sudden or slowly lingering).

Material

From the total group of 338 patients (cf. Part I) a group of 23 cases (19 females and 4 males) with pronounced functional symptoms was selected. These patients were subjected to a thorough clinical examination, only persons with no signs of somatic disorders being selected.

23 normal subjects, age- and sex-matched to the group of patients, formed a control group. The controls were examined in the same manner as the patients.

Results

On MCT most patients (n = 19) but only few controls (n = 5) show signs of free-floating anxiety (p < 0.00025).

The primary aim in using the SAE in the present study was to consider the different patterns in relation to the patients' reports of their dizziness as either a turning sensation inside the head or a spinning sensation outside the head. Thereby patients with a hysteric SAE style (short durations), which also implies *highly extraverted* behavior, were expected to locate their dizziness as being outside the head. Patients with other SAE patterns were expected to more often report their dizziness as being inside the head. There were 7 patients with a hysteric SAE style. Most patients (n = 5) with a hysteric SAE style located their dizziness as being outside the head, while patients with other SAE patterns more often reported their dizziness as being inside the head (p = 0.021).

Table I. Differing characteristics of patients in the two subgroups

Instrument	Hysteric vertigo patients	Obsessional vertigo patients	p value
MCT	less signs of anxiety	more signs of anxiety	0.13
Questionnaire	no functional symptoms before dizziness	functional symptoms before dizziness	0.013
Questionnaire	first dizziness sensation slowly lingering	first dizziness sensation sudden and linked up with a precise event	0.013

These results suggest two different types of psychogenic vertigo patients. It was possible, by combining the findings on SAE and MCT, to classify 21 of the 23 patients into two nonoverlapping subgroups. One group (n = 13) was characterized by signs of repression (hysteria) on MCT and/or a hysteric style on SAE, the other (n = 8) by signs of isolation (obsessional neurosis) on MCT. From table I it is clear that the two groups of psychogenic vertigo patients differ in several respects.

From a clinical point of view we also find it notable that a follow-up 2 years after the psychological investigation reveals continuing differences between the two patient groups concerning their dizziness symptoms. Most hysteric vertigo patients (n = 10) rate themselves as improved (only 1 patient reports that the dizziness has disappeared), while 6 obsessional vertigo patients report their dizziness as nonimproved (1 patient reported it as having worsened) (p = 0.03). Since the patients' treatment consisted mainly in taking tranquilizers, a tentative interpretation of the follow-up results is that such treatment is more effective with hysteric psychogenic vertigo patients. However, in vertigo patients showing signs of obsessional tendencies combined with a more marked proneness for manifest anxiety (table I), such treatment is less relevant. These findings, we think, are important to bear in mind in selecting therapeutic measures for the psychogenic vertigo patient.

Nervous vertigo and dizziness may thus be a rather common symptom. In spite of this we may assume that these patients do not yet attract proper attention neither by otologists nor by psychiatrists. The reasons for this may be many. The otologists may have little understanding of nervousness and the psychiatrists may be scared by the possibility of a somatic source of the vertigo or dizziness. This results in a large number of nervous and vertiginous patients are left alone without medical assistance with their scaring and invalidating symptoms.

References

Afzelius, L.-E.: Yrsel – en klinisk analys; thesis Lund (1975).

Afzelius, L.-E.; Henriksson, N.G., and Wahlgren, L.: Vertigo and dizziness of functional origin (accepted for publication, 1978).

Andersson, A.L.; Nilsson, A., and Henriksson, N.G.: Personality differences between accident-loaded and accident-free young car drivers. Br. J. Psychol. *61:* 409–421 (1970).

Andersson, A.L.; Nilsson, A.; Ruuth, E., and Smith, G.J.W.: Visual aftereffects and the individual as an adaptive system (Gleerup, Lund 1972).

Henriksson, N.G. and Afzelius, L.-E.: Effect of eye-closure on vestibular nystagmus reflecting alertness and personality. Suppl. Int. J. Equil. Res. (1975).

Henriksson, N.G.; Afzelius, L.-E., and Wahlgren, L.: Vertigo and rocking sensation. ORL *38:* 206–217 (1976).

Magnusson, P.-Å.; Nilsson, A., and Henriksson, N.G.: Psychogenic vertigo within an anxiety frame of reference: an experimental study. Br. J. med. Psychol. *50:* 187–201 (1977).

Nilsson, A.: Adaptive and defensive aspects of the individual: a system approach to adaptation in relationship to a psychoanalytic anxiety model. Int. Rev. Psycho-Anal. *4:* 111–123 (1977).

Sloane, P.: Psychiatric aspects of vertigo; in Spector, Dizziness and vertigo, pp. 258–262 (Grune & Stratton, New York 1967).

Smith, G.J.W.; Johnson, G.; Ljunghill-Andersson, J., and Almgren, P.E.: MCT-meta-kontrasttekniken (Skand. Testförlaget, Stockholm 1970).

N.G. Henriksson, MD, University Hospital of Lund,
Department of Otorhinolaryngology, Lund (Sweden)

Adv. Oto-Rhino-Laryng., vol. 25, pp. 100–105 (Karger, Basel 1979)

Meniere's Disease: a Neuropsychological Study II

K. Zilstorff, J. Thomsen, P. Laursen, G. Hoffmann, O. Kjærby,
B. Paludan and A. Theilgaard

ENT Department and Department of Psychiatry, University of Copenhagen,
Rigshospitalet, Copenhagen

Introduction

Since 1950 a substantial amount of research on the psychopathological aspects of Meniere's disease has been carried out.

Löchen [1970] studied the neuropsychological functions in 30 patients with Meniere's disease. *Löchen* compared the Meniere patients with patients who suffered from severe cerebral atrophy and demonstrated that all Meniere patients had pathological neurologic and/or pneumoencephalographic traits, besides neuropsychological disturbances. The average age was about 50 years. The duration of the disease for the 30 patients was not reported.

Crary et al. [1976] has criticized the validity of these findings and claim that *Löchen's* [1970] results do not include statistically significant discrepancies between Meniere patients and the normal population, if age-equivalence, as used in the WAIS-age distribution figures (i.e. Wechsler Adult Intelligence Scales), is taken into consideration. In their study, *Crary et al.* [1976] compared Meniere patients with patients who suffered from other forms of otologic illnesses. The neuropsychologic test results showed no differences between the groups, and on the basis of this, *Crary et al.* [1976] rejects the hypothesis of cerebral changes appearing as a clinical factor in Meniere's disease.

More personality-oriented psychological studies were first proposed by *Fowler and Zeckel* in 1952 and later in 1953. They proposed a psychosomatic etiology for Meniere's disease as a possibility. This hypothesis has been sought and supported by others [e.g. *Siirala et al.,* 1965; *Hinchcliffe,* 1967; *Williamsen and Giffort,* 1971; *Stephens,* 1975]. However, e.g., *Watson et al.* [1967] and *Pulec and House* [1973] arrived at results which contradicted this theory.

Hinchcliffe [1967] discussed two alternative hypothesis: (1) that the psychological disturbances were secondary to the vestibular disorders (i.e. somatopsychic effect), and (2) that the psychological disturbances were primary to the vestibular disorders (i.e. psychosomatic effect). In referring to several investigators, *Hinchcliffe* [1967] concluded that both hypotheses are upheld, but that the MMPI method (Minnesota Multiphasic Personality Inventory) has shown an increased prevalence of psychosomatic type of personality profiles in patients with Meniere's disease, as compared with a control population (otosclerosis).

Kirkegaard Sørensen et al. [1977] studied a group of 19 Meniere patients to establish whether localization of the hearing reduction and vestibular changes have any relation to the lateralization of a possible organic dysfunction. This study of patients having Meniere's disease for an average duration of 10 years, demonstrated that right-handed patients with defect hearing in the left ear evidenced an organic dysfunction, reflecting a deficit of long-term memory of visual material, in verbal abstraction and learning of mazes. The study indicated no general intellectual deficit, but the results indicated that patients with defect hearing in left ear might have a disturbance in functions presumably represented in the nondominant hemisphere. It was suggested that lesions in Meniere's disease may not be entirely peripheral and that the neuropsychological disturbances are secondary to a peripheral acousticovestibular disorder.

In selecting the tests for our present investigation it was considered that the results should give quantitative data which could be treated by statistical methods. In addition we wanted to study a wide range of cognitive functions. These were learning, memory, abstraction, activation of goal-directed behavior. We also found it important to estimate the hand preference and the premorbid intelligence level. To clarify the question of lateralization of the dysfunction, easy-to-verbalize (verbal) tests, presumably representing functions in left vs. right hemisphere in right-handed persons were also included.

Method

The subject group consists of 23 outpatients with Meniere's disease – 8 females and 15 males, age range 29–70 years and mean age of 51,4 years. According to *Oldfield*'s [1971] hand-preference list, all subjects are right-handed. The majority of subjects have

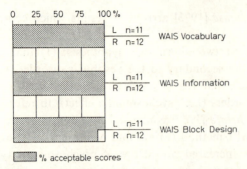

Fig. 1. Results of vocabulary, information and block design subtests from the WAIS (Wechsler Adult Intelligence Scales), showing normal intelligence for all the patients. L=Left ear hearing defect; R=right ear hearing defect.

relative low socioeconomic status on a scale of 1–5 [*Svalastoga,* 1959], 18 subjects obtain a score of 4 and/or below.

The subjects have been tested with an extensive neuropsychological test battery, including Vocabulary, Information and Block Design tests from the WAIS [*Wechsler,* 1955], Stroop Color Naming Test, Face Recognition, RA Visual Gestalts, Paired Associates, Sentence Reproduction and Rod & Frame Test. These tests are described in detail elsewhere [*Zilstorff et al.,* 1979].

Results

In view of the absence of controls the patients' scores are compared with norms obtained from normal groups. The patients are divided into those with left and those with right hearing defects. The size of the material does not allow for further separating the patients into age and sex groups.

The percentage of patients with acceptable scores, e.g. scores within the normal distribution, is indicated by black columns in the figures. It appears, judging from the results of the three subtests of WAIS, that the general intelligence level for the entire group is within normal limits (fig. 1).

Memory as reflected by Word Pairs and Visual Gestalts is compromised for patients with left as well as with right hearing defects. The learning phase seems more compromised than the reproduction phase, and the group of patients with right hearing defect show the greatest deviation from normal results (fig. 2). Almost all patients manage the sentence completion, but again the right hearing defect group is inferior to the left one (fig. 3).

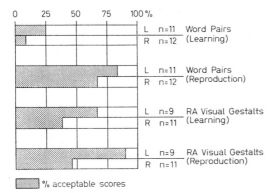

Fig. 2. Results of Word Pairs and Visual Gestalts, testing memory, showing poor performance, the learning phase seeming more compromised than the reproduction phase.

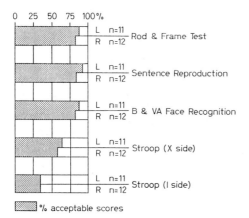

Fig. 3. Results of the Rod and Frame test, testing cognitive style or intellectual performance, showing normal values. Sentence reproduction, testing short-time memory, showing normal values. B & VA Face Recognition, presumably testing right hemisphere, showing normal values. Results of Stroop Color Naming test, testing concentration, showing poor performance.

Attention (Stroop) is the function which next to verbal learning presents the greatest problem to the patients. There is no essential difference with regard to laterality of hearing defect (fig. 3).

Discussion

The patient material in this study is similar to the group we studied previously [*Kirkegaard et al.,* 1977] with regard to size, age distribution and socioeconomic level, but differs in the essential aspect of duration of illness. This present study deals with patients with a recent debut of Meniere's disease (approx. 1 year) whereas the former study included patients with long-range manifestation of Meniere's disease (average 10 years). The present study includes almost twice as many men as women, whereas the first investigation presented a 1:1 ratio in sex distribution.

No signs of general intellectual impairment were found in either study, and weakness of concentration is a common feature found in both materials. A dysfunction of memory is also evidenced in the present group, but contrary to the first study, material specificity did not influence the results.

There is no statistically significant difference between the groups with right and left ear hearing defects, contrary to the findings of the former study, but the right hearing defect group shows a tendency to poorer performance, especially in learning of Visual Gestalts and Word Pairs.

Discrepancy of the results in the two studies with regard to laterality i.e. the different hemisphere function, might be due to the small sample size, or more probably to the fact that illness duration of studies sample is 1 year opposed to 10 years of the former studies group, so that the central changes in the nondominant hemisphere function demonstrated in the first study develop over a long period of time.

We hope further neuropsychological investigations of Meniere patients can give us more information of what is primary in Meniere's disease: peripheral sensory or central neurological changes.

Summary

23 Meniere patients were examined with an extensive battery of neuropsychological tests. In a previous investigation the authors had demonstrated that patients with a long duration of Meniere's disease had psychological disturbances, presumably localized in the nondominant hemisphere. In the present investigation the patients had a short duration of the disease, and we were unable to reproduce the psychological disturbances. It is concluded that the central changes in the nondominant hemisphere function develop over a long period of time. It is hoped for that further neuropsychological investigations of Meniere patients can give more information of what is primary in Meniere's disease: peripheral sensory or central neurological changes.

References

Crary, G.; Wexler, M., and Ribey, A.: Meniere's disease and cerebral impairment. Archs. Otolar. *102:* 368 (1976).

Fowler, E.P. and Zeckel, A.: Psychosomatic aspects of Meniere's disease. Psychosom. Med. *14:* 1265 (1952).

Fowler, E.P. and Zeckel, A.: Psychophysiological factors in Meniere's disease. Psychosom. Med. *15:* 127 (1953).

Hinchcliffe, R.: Personality profile in Meniere's disease. J. Lar. Otol. *81:* 476 (1967).

Kirkegaard Sørensen, L.; Theilgaard, A.; Thomsen, J., and Zilstorff, K.: Meniere's disease A neuropsychological study. Acta oto-lar. *83:* 266 (1977).

Löchen, E.A.: Morbus meniere. A complexity of pathological manifestation. Acta neurol. scand. *46:* suppl., p. 5 (1970).

Oldfield, R.C.: The assessment and analysis of handedness: The Edinburgh Inventory. Neuropsychologia *9:* 97 (1971).

Pulec, L. and House, W.F.: Meniere's disease study. Three-year progress report. Equilibrium Res. *3:* 156 (1973).

Siirala, U.; Siltala, P., and Lumio, J.S.: Psychological aspects of Meniere's disease. Acta oto-lar. *59:* 350 (1965).

Stephens, S.D.G.: Personality tests in Meniere's disorder. J. Laryng. *89:* 479 (1975).

Svalastoga, K.: Prestige, class and mobility (Gyldendal, København 1959).

Watson, C.G.; Barnes, C.; Donaldson, J.A., and Klett, W.G.: Psychosomatic aspects of Meniere's disease. Acta oto-lar. *86:* 543 (1967).

Wechsler, D.: Manual for the Wechsler Adult Intelligence Scale. (The Psychological Cooperation, New York 1955).

Williamsen, D.G. and Giffort, F.: Psychosomatic aspects of Meniere's disease. Acta oto-lar. *72:* 118 (1971).

Zilstorff, K.; Thomsen, J.; Laursen, P.; Hoffmann, G.; Kjærby, O.; Paludan, B., and Theilgaard, A.: Meniere's disease. A neuropsychological study II. ORL (in press, 1979).

Kaj Zilstorff, MD, University ENT Department Rigshospitalet, Blegdamsvej 9, DK-2100 Copenhagen (Denmark)

Adv. Oto-Rhino-Laryng., vol. 25, pp. 106–111 (Karger, Basel 1979)

Epidemiological Survey of Definite Cases of Meniere's Disease Collected by the Seventeen Members of the Meniere's Disease Research Committee of Japan in 1975–1976[1]

K. Mizukoshi, H. Ino, K. Ishikawa, Y. Watanabe, H. Yamazaki, I. Kato, J. Okubo and I. Watanabe

Department of Otolaryngology, Niigata University School of Medicine, Niigata, Department of Otolaryngology, Yamagata University School of Medicine, Yamagata, and Department of Otolaryngology, Tokyo Medical and Dental University, Tokyo

Introduction

A number of studies of Meniere's disease have been reported in Japan during the past 20 years. However, these studies were based on observations of a relatively small number of cases collected from a limited number of otolaryngologists. In 1974, the Meniere's Disease Research Committee of Japan, which is supported by the Ministry of Health and Welfare, was founded by 17 doctors [5]. These doctors, who are distributed between the epidemiological, clinical and etiological research sections of the Committee, come from various districts or areas of Japan.

In the first survey, 580 cases of definite Meniere's disease were collected from the 17 members of the Committee during the period January 1973 to December 1974. This epidemiological survey was reported by *Watanabe et al.* [6]. Then, between April 1975 and December 1976, the second nationwide survey was carried out by the same members.

Materials and Methods

In order to collect as many of the same cases of definite Meniere's disease as possible, the Committee drafted the diagnostic criteria of the disease reported by *Watanabe* [5].

[1] This work was supported by a grant from the Ministry of Health and Welfare, Japan.

In the second nationwide survey, the epidemiological and clinical data from 520 patients with definite Meniere's disease were collected from the 17 members of the Committee by using a data-processing sheet containing questionnaires. In order to make a control study of definite Meniere's disease, details of 126 patients with non-Meniere vertigo and/or dizziness (Control A), in whom Meniere's disease had been ruled out by neuro-otological assessments, and 288 patients with rhinolaryngological disorders (Control B) were collected in the same way. These epidemiological data were stored and analyzed by a PDP 11/40 computer.

Results and Comments

The characteristic epidemiological features in the second nationwide survey of definite cases of Meniere's disease in Japan have been classified according to three groups of factors, i.e., individual factors, environmental factors and original-occurrence factors.

Individual Factors (Personal Factors)

Sex Ratio. The sex ratio and the age distribution at onset in the definite cases of Meniere's disease are represented in table I. The male:female ratio

Table I. Sex ratio and age distribution at onset in 520 cases of definite Meniere's disease collected from the 17 members of the Meniere's Disease Research Committee of Japan (1975–1976)

Age	Meniere's disease							
	definite				suspected			
	male		female		male		female	
	n	%	n	%	n	%	n	%
–9	0	0	1	0.4	1	1.7	0	0
10–19	12	4.7	14	5.5	0	0	3	2.7
20–29	36	14.1	34	13.3	12	20.3	17	15.0
30–39	65	25.5	72	28.2	15	25.4	39	34.6
40–49	88	34.5	64	25.1	18	30.5	31	27.4
50–59	34	13.3	52	20.4	8	13.6	18	15.9
60–69	15	5.9	16	6.3	5	8.5	5	4.4
70–79	4	1.6	2	0.8	0	0	0	0
80–	1	0.4	0	0	0	0	0	0
Total	255	100	255	100	59	100	113	100
Unknown	4		6		0		0	

in these cases was almost the same. On the other hand, the ratio of suspected cases was lower in males than in females.

Age Distribution at Onset. The age distribution of patients with definite Meniere's disease peaks at the age group of 40–49 years for males, while the peak for females is at the age group of 30–39 years. However, in both control groups, A and B, the sex ratio and the age distribution were shown to be similar to those for the Meniere's disease series.

Personality Characteristics. The personalities of the patients with Meniere's disease were evaluated by using Miyagi's Questionnaire. In the patients with definite Meniere's disease, neurosis and precisianism were frequently observed. However, there were no significant personality differences between the patients in the Meniere's disease series and those in the control series.

Family History. 5.8% of the 520 patients with definite Meniere's disease had a close relative who also suffered from Meniere's disease. On the other hand, the control groups had increased rates of family cases.

Marriage. There was a higher incidence of definite Meniere's disease in married persons (85.7%) than in the two control groups, A and B.

Drinking and Smoking. There was no apparent relationship between the onset of definite Meniere's disease and drinking and/or smoking.

Environmental Factors
Annual Distribution. According to *Nakae and Komatsuzaki* [3], the annual ratio of patients with Meniere's disease to the total annual number of outpatients has been constant since about 1964, although the ratio of suspected cases has varied.

Season and Time of Onset. There was no seasonal variation in onset in the definite cases of Meniere's disease. On the other hand, there was a high frequency of initial vertiginous attacks in the morning and in the afternoon in these cases.

Geographical Distribution. The geographical distribution of definite cases of Meniere's disease was also noted in this survey. There was an increasing number of cases in the southern area of the Kanto district, compared with the northern area. This tendency has already been reported by *Naito* [2] and *Watanabe et al.* [6].

Occupational Distribution. There was an apparently higher incidence of definite cases of Meniere's disease among technicians than among farmers, fishermen and laborers engaged in simple work.

Noisy Environment. There was no apparent relationship between the onset of definite Meniere's disease and a noisy environment.

Original-Occurrence Factors
Past Medical History. There was no apparent, special, past medical history in the definite cases of Meniere's disease.

Complications. There were no special complications in the cases of definite Meniere's disease, except for hypotension (6.3%).

Preceding Events. Mental and physical fatigue before vertiginous attacts were reported in 35.0 and 33.3% of the cases of definite Meniere's disease respectively, figures which were significantly higher than those in the control series.

Condition at the Initial Vertiginous Attacks. There was a high incidence of onset when getting up in the morning (21.2%), when working (21.9%) and when housekeeping (10.6%).

Initial Symptoms. The frequency of initial symptoms at the onset of vertiginous attacks in the cases of definite Meniere's disease was noted. These symptoms were more frequent in the group of patients with onset of cochlear signs before vertigo (66.7%) than in the group of patients with onset of cochlear and vertiginous signs together (28.7%) and with vertigo noticed before the cochlear signs (5.2%). These features were different from those observed in the first nationwide survey [6].

In considering these data, it may appear that the occurrence of vertiginous attacks in cases of Meniere's disease is influenced more by individual than by environmental factors. However, this feature can be considered as another evidence of the psychosomatic disorders involved in Meniere's disease [1].

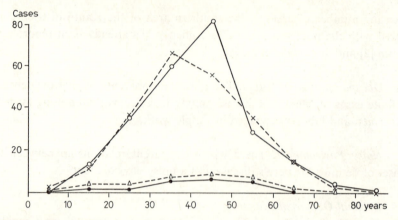

Fig. 1. Sex ratio and age distribution at onset in 472 cases of unilateral (○ = male; × = female) Meniere's disease and in 48 cases of bilateral (● = male; △ = female) Meniere's disease (1975–1976).

Finally, when an estimate was made concerning the affected side in the cases of Meniere's disease on the bases of the clinical symptomatology, 48 (9.2%) of the 520 patients were found to have bilateral Meniere's disease. The sex ratio and the age distribution of bilateral Meniere's disease are shown in figure 1. The male:female ratio of bilateral Meniere's disease was 66:100. The female preponderance was more marked than that in cases of unilateral Meniere's disease. Moreover, our statistical data indicate that the incidence of bilateral Meniere's disease increases with the duration of the disease. These features are in accordance with those described by *Stahle* [4].

Summary

Between April 1975 and December 1976, the second nationwide survey of Meniere's disease in Japan was made by the 17 members of the Meniere's Disease Research Committee of Japan. The epidemiological data from 520 patients with definite Meniere's disease were analyzed in comparison with those from the 126 patients in the non-Meniere vertiginous group (Control A) and the 228 patients in the rhinolaryngological group (Control B).

The male:female ratio of definite cases of Meniere's disease was almost the same, and the age distribution peaked at the age group of 40–49 years for males, while the peak for females was at the age group of 30–39 years. 5.8% of the 520 patients had a close relative who also suffered from Meniere's disease. From the epidemiological features, it may appear that the occurrence of vertiginous attacks in Meniere's disease is influenced much more by individual than by environmental factors. However, this feature can be considered as another evidence of the psychosomatic disorders involved in Meniere's disease.

References

1   Hinchcliffe, R.: Personal and family medical history in Meniere's disease. J. Lar. Otol. *81:* 661–668 (1967).
2   Naito, T.: Recent studies on Meniere's disease. Pract. Otol., Kyoto *66:* suppl., pp. 1–48 (1973).
3   Nakae, K. and Komatsuzaki, A.: Epidemiological study of Meniere's disease. Pract. Otol., Kyoto *69:* 1783–1788 (1976).
4   Stahle, J.: Advanced Meniere's disease: a study of 356 severely disabled patients. Acta oto-lar. *81:* 113–119 (1976).
5   Watanabe, I.: Meniere's Disease Research Committee of Japan; in Morimoto, Proc. 5th Extraordinary Meeting of the Barany Society in Kyoto, 1975. Int. J. Equilibrium Res. suppl., pp. 281–283 (1976).
6   Watanabe, I.; Okubo, J.; Mizukoshi, K., and Nakae, K.: Result of epidemiological investigation of definite cases of Meniere's disease collected from seventeen hospitals in various locations in Japan. Pract. Otol., Kyoto *69:* 1776–1782 (1976).

K. Mizukoshi, MD, Department of Otolaryngology, Niigata University, School of Medicine, Asahi-Machi 1, Niigata 951 (Japan)

Adv. Oto-Rhino-Laryng., vol. 25, pp. 112–116 (Karger, Basel 1979)

Neurotological Studies on Meniere's Disease and Sudden Deafness[1]

H. Ino, K. Mizukoshi, K. Ishikawa, Y. Watanabe, H. Yamazaki, M. Aoyagi and I. Kato

Department of Otolaryngology, Niigata University School of Medicine, Niigata and Department of Otolaryngology, Yamagata University School of Medicine, Yamagata

Introduction

In 1973 and 1974, it was decided by the Ministry of Health and Welfare, Japan, that sudden deafness and Meniere's disease should be investigated as a 'specific disease' respectively. Nationwide and concentrated epidemiological, clinical and etiological researches are now carried out on Meniere's disease. It is well known that the onset of sudden deafness is often accompanied with vertigo, which is a very similar symptom to Meniere's disease. Moreover, clinical differential diagnosis of both diseases at the early stage is necessary for adequate and proper treatment. However, few reports have dealt with the relationship between Meniere's disease and sudden deafness. Therefore, we tried a neurotological assessment for two types of diseases each and compared the characteristic signs and symptoms with special reference to neurotological findings.

Materials and Methods

Among all outpatients whom we examined and who complained of vertigo or dizziness and sudden onset of hearing impairment from January 1973 to June 1975 at the Department of Otolaryngology, Niigata University School of Medicine, in Niigata, 60 cases with definite Meniere's disease and 30 cases with sudden deafness were listed according to such criteria for the diagnosis of both diseases as determined by the Research Committee. In Meniere's disease series, 27 males and 33 females were tested, while 15 males and 15 females with sudden deafness were also tested. The diagnostic criteria for

[1] Supported by a grant from the Ministry of Health and Welfare.

Table I. Diagnostic criteria of sudded deafness (Sudden Deafness Research Committee of Japan, 1973)

Condition
I Main symptoms
   1 Hearing impairment of sudden onset
   2 Severe sensory hearing loss
   3 Origin of the hearing loss is unknown
II Associated symtoms
   1 In most cases, hearing impairment associated with tinnitus at the time of onset
   2 In some cases, these hearing impairments associated with single vertiginous attack or unsteady feeling in the early stage
   3 Exclusion of central nervous system disorders

Diagnostic criteria
   1 Definite cases: conformable to all of conditions I and II
   2 Suspicious cases: conformable to I, 1 and 2

Meniere's disease were applied to our cases with definite Meniere's disease, which were reported by *Watanabe* [5]. On the other hand, the diagnostic criteria for sudden deafness were applied to all patients with sudden hearing impairment, which were represented in table I.

The neurotological examinations routinely employed during the period from 1973 to 1976 are listed as follows: (a) *Audiometry:* (1) pure tone audiometry; (2) speech audiometry; (3) audiological recruitment test: ABLB, SISI, Metz's recruitment test by stapedius reflex, and (4) Bekesy's audiometry; (b) *Equilibrium test:* (1) spontaneous nystagmus (Gaze nystagmus; observed with Frenzel's spectacles and ENG); (2) positional nystagmus test, (3) experimental nystagmus test: caloric nystagmus (hot-cold irrigation), optokinetic nystagmus (horizontal and vertical stimuli with constant acceleration), eye-tracking test (ETT, horizontal and vertical sinusoidal smooth pursuits), and (4) Fukuda's stepping test and Mann's test.

All the eye movements were recorded by means of ENG and were evaluated by the normal values of caloric nystagmus and optokinetic nystagmus, as determined by *Ohtani* [3] and *Ino* [1]. The test methods and procedures were also followed by those of *Mizukoshi et al.* [2].

Results and Comments

Neurotological signs and symptoms obtained from our observations were as follows.

Subjective Signs and Symptoms. At the early stage, definite Meniere's disease was characterized by spontaneous (95%), paroxysmal (98%), recurrent (100%), and vertiginous attacks (92%) accompanied by cochlear

Table II. Hearing impairment observed in the cases with 'definite' Meniere's disease and in these with sudden deafness

Pure tone loss, dB (pure tone average) (a+2b+c/4)	Meniere's disease (88 ears)		Sudden deafness (31 ears)	
	n	%	n	%
1 0–19	24	32	0	0
2 20–39	19	26	2	6
3 40–59	21	28	6	19
4 60–79	9	12	9	29
5 80–	1	1.4	14	47

signs such as tinnitus (93%), hearing loss (73%), and nausea and/or vomiting (75%) in our 60 cases series. On the other hand, the nature of vertigo observed in 30 cases with sudden deafness was provoked (40%) as well as spontaneous (32%) and paroxysmal (88%), while single vertiginous attacks (56%) with hearing impairments (100%) were much more commonly observed. In general, about half of the patients with sudden deafness did not remember having had any vertiginous symptoms. However, in 83% of our patients, associated vertigo was recognized at the onset of sudden deafness. The reason for this is that many of the patients in our series were examined for dysequilibrium at the recovery stage as well as at the later stage.

Audiological Findings. In patients with definite Meniere's disease, hearing impairment was generally slight and characterized by deficiency in detecting low- and middle-pitched tones: the pure tone audiograms revealed the flat curve (32%), the rising curve (28%), the falling curve (13%) and the mountain curve (22%) in this series.

The distribution of the patients with both diseases on the basis of the mean value of hearing threshold are shown in table II. Sudden deafness was characterized by highly impaired hearing, i.e., total deafness was observed in 14 cases (45%).

Fluctuation of auditory threshold was observed in 42 cases (70%), regardless of the course in definite Meniere's disease, and much common in the low frequency range. In sudden deafness, on the contrary, hearing impairment tended to improve in all frequency ranges. In definite Meniere's disease, recruitment phenomena as shown by the ABLB, SISI, Bekesy's

Table III. Relationship between the affected sides and the nystagmus findings observed in the cases with Meniere's disease and in these with sudden deafness

Nystagmus findings	Meniere's Disease (60)		Sudden deafness (30)	
	toward the affected side	toward the intact side	toward the affected side	toward the intact side
1 Spontaneous nystagmus	21	14	9	11
2 Caloric nystagmus				
1 CP	23	0	11	0
2 Hyperexcitability	2	0		
3 Direction of DP	13	9	2	4
4 Bilateral hypofunction	3	3	2	2
5 Normal	9	9	9	9

audiometry and Metz's Recruitment test by stapedius reflex were positive in 20 (80%) out of 25 cases tested. In sudden deafness, the same recruitment phenomena were recognized in 8 (80%) of 10 cases tested, but the hearing impairment of retrocochlear type was observed as type III by Bekesy's audiometry in only 1 case.

Equilibrium Findings. Spontaneous nystagmus in Meniere's disease series was observed in 39 cases (65%) on ENG during mental arithmetic with the eyes closed, and positional nystagmus was also observed in 82%. In 20 (67%) of 30 cases with sudden deafness, on the other hand, spontaneous nystagmus was observed on ENG, and positional nystagmus was also recorded in 20 cases (67%), regardless of associated vertigo. In the experimental nystagmus tests, abnormal caloric responses such as CP (canal paresis) and DP (directional preponderance) were observed in 51 cases (85%), and CP of the affected ears was also observed in 26 cases (43%) with definite Meniere's diseases. In the sudden deafness series, abnormal caloric responses were observed in 20 cases (67%) regardless of associated vertigo, and CP of the affected ears was also observed in 11 cases (37%). However, abnormal optokinetic nystagmus and/or eye-tracking were observed in only 9 cases (19%) with definite Meniere's disease, and were also observed in 8 cases (27%) with sudden deafness.

When ENG recording were compared between definite Meniere's disease and sudden deafness, it was found that the incidence of spontaneous nystagmus was nearly the same regardless of associated vertigo and the course of both diseases. Moreover, estimation based on symptomatology was made of the affected side in both diseases and a relationship between the affected side and the nystagmus findings were summarized in table III. The direction of spontaneous nystagmus and the directional preponderance of caloric nystagmus appeared to have no definite correlation with the affected side in both Meniere's disease and sudden deafness. However, it was also reconfirmed that a reduction in caloric nystagmus was a better indicator for assessment of the affected ear.

Moreover, hyperexcitability in caloric nystagmus was noted in only 2 cases with Meniere's disease, in accordance with previous observations [4].

Summary

During the period from January 1973 to June 1975, 60 cases with definite Meniere's disease and 30 cases with sudden deafness were listed according to such criteria for the diagnosis of both diseases as determined by the Research Committee of Japan. A neuro-otological assessment for both diseases was performed in our series. In patients with definite Meniere's disease, hearing impairment was characterized by deficiency in detecting low- and middle-pitched tones and fluctuation of auditory threshold in low frequency range. In sudden deafness, highly impaired hearing loss, i.e., total deafness, was frequently observed (45%). However, recruitment occurred at the same incidence (80%) in both diseases tested. The incidence of spontaneous nystagmus was almost the same regardless of associated vertigo and the course of both diseases. Moreover, it was also recognized that a reduction of caloric responses was a better indication for assessment of the affected ear in both diseases.

References

1   Ino, H.: Optokinetic nystagmus; in Stahle, Vestibular function on earth and in space, pp. 209–214 (Pergamon Press, Oxford 1970).
2   Mizukoshi, K;. Nagaba, M.; Ohno, Y.; Ishikawa, K.; Aoyagi, M.; Watanabe, Y.; Kato, I., and Ino, H.: Neurotological studies upon intoxication by organic mercury compounds. ORL 37: 74–87 (1975).
3   Ohtani, T.: Which is the best value to estimate the vestibular function? Jap. J. Otol., Tokyo 65: 524–543 (1962).
4   Stahle, J.: Advanced Meniere's disease: a study of 356 severely disabled patients. Acta oto-lar. 81: 113–119 (1976).
5   Watanabe, I.: Meniere's Disease Research Committee of Japan; in Morimoto, Proc. 5th Extraord. Meet. Barany Society, Kyoto 1975. Int. J. Equilibrium Res., suppl. pp. 281–283 (1976).

Hatsuo Ino, MD, Department of Otolaryngology,
Niigata University School of Medicine, Niigata (Japan)

Adv. Oto-Rhino-Laryng., vol. 25, pp. 117–121 (Karger, Basel 1979)

Bilateral Meniere's Disease

M. Kitahara, H. Matsubara, T. Takeda and Y. Yazawa

Department of Otolaryngology (Head: Prof. *M. Kitahara*),
Shiga University of Medical Science, Otsu

Introduction

Although bilateral involvement of Meniere's disease is serious enough to produce a high degree of deafness in both ears, actually little attention has been directed to such involvement.

In the literature, even the incidence of bilateral involvement shows a wide variation from 2 to 78%. Also the somatic and psychiatric aspects of bilateral Meniere's disease remain to be elucidated. In this paper, the characteristic feature of bilateral involvement in Meniere's disease are discussed in comparision with unilateral involvement, and the clinical management is outlined.

Material and Methods

A survey was conducted on 265 Japanese patients with Meniere's disease who were treated at the clinic of the Department of Otolaryngology, Faculty of Medicine, Kyoto University. The group consisted of 113 males and 152 females. Diagnosis of Meniere's disease was limited to patients with recurrent attacks of idiopathic vertigo, sensory-neural deafness and/or tinnitus in episodic relationship. In this investigation, all patients were questioned carefully as to whether they had experienced tinnitus and/or deafness in the contralateral ear during vertiginous attack. As the attention of the patients with Meniere's disease was concentrated on the vertiginous attack itself, they were often unaware of slight tinnitus and/or deafness in the contralateral ear. This was particularly so in cases involving aggravation of tinnitus and/or deafness simultaneously in both ears. Glycerol and furosemide tests and electrocochleographic studies were also conducted when necessary, since the evaluation of recruitment is most difficult in cases of bilateral involvement. Glycerol and furosemide tests were done according to Klockhoff's method and Kitahara and Futaki's method, respectively. The electrocochleogram was recorded through a metal skin surface electrode with an acoustic click stimuli. Patients with a ratio of the amplitude of the summating potential (SP) to the compound action potential (AP) of the cochlear nerve, of more than 0.37, under a click intensity of 105 dB pe SPL, were diagnosed as having Meniere's disease.

Results

Bilateral involvement was found in 29% or 78 of the 265 patients with Meniere's disease. This group included 33 males and 45 females, while unilateral involvement included 88 males and 107 females. Here the distribution was not significantly different between these two groups. The onset of the disease in 84% of the patients was between the ages of 20 and 60 years. Patients who were over 60 at the onset of the disease included 14.1% of the bilateral cases, while the rate was 4.9% in cases of unilateral involvement. That is, there was often bilateral involvement when the onset occurred in persons of an advanced age. Somatic and psychiatric aspects of bilateral Meniere's disease were as follows:

Duration of the Disease and Frequency of Attacks

Patients who had had the disease for 10 years or more accounted for 21.8% of the bilateral cases, while the rate was 11.0% in cases of unilateral involvement. That is, the duration of the disease in cases of bilateral involvement was significantly longer than unilateral involvement, as was also reported by *Enander and Stahle* [2]. Regarding the frequency of attacks, no differences were observed between the two groups.

Audiological Investigation

The distribution of hearing loss in the ears with a lesser degree of deafness in bilateral cases was not significantly different from that of unilateral cases. A sensorineural loss of more than 60 dB was observed in 33.4% of ears with a more intensive degree of deafness in bilateral cases and in 11.9% of unilateral cases. That is, the hearing loss of ears with a more intensive degree of deafness in bilateral cases was significantly more severe as compared with that of unilateral involvement. In other words, in cases of bilateral involvement, a more extensive degree of hearing loss was frequently diagnosed. In this study, the degree of hearing loss was calculated from the mean value of the air conduction at a frequency of 500, 1,000 and 2,000 Hz. Regarding the distribution of the configuration which was

sparse, flattened endothelium remained. In the 4 patients with long-standing Meniere's disease and some permanent loss of auditory and vestibular function, the lumen of the sac could not be identified histologically, even though a 'lumen' was thought to be visible to the surgeon at the time of endolymphatic sac biopsy and decompression. The lack of correlation between the surgeon's observation and histologic verification of the endolymphatic sac lumen in long-standing Meniere's disease suggests that accurate placement of drainage tubes in the lumen of the endolymphatic sac can be very problematical.

Summary

Biopsies of the endolymphatic sac were performed in 6 patients undergoing endolymphatic sac decompression and/or drainage procedures. Electron microscopy revealed extensive subendothelial fibrosis with loss of vascularity, heavy deposition of collagen and flattening of luminal cells. In patients with long-standing disease, complete obliteration of the endolymphatic sac lumen appeared to occur. There was poor correlation between the surgeon's ability to identify the lumen of the endolymphatic sac and its presence in the biopsy specimen.

References

1   Hallpike, C.S. and Cairns, H.: Observations on the pathology of Meniere's syndrome. Proc. R. Soc. Med. *31:* 1317–1336 (1938).
2   Portmann, G.: Recherches sur le sac endolymphatique: résultats et applications chirurgicales. Acta oto-lar. *11:* 110–137 (1927).
3   Guild, S.R.: The circulation of endolymph. Am. J. Anat. *39:* 57–81 (1927).
4   Wittmaack, K.: Die Ortho- und Pathobiologie des Labyrinthes (Thieme, Stuttgart 1956).
5   Altman, F. and Fowler, E.P., jr.: Histologic findings in Meniere's symptom complex. Ann. Otol. Rhinol. Lar. *52:* 52–80 (1943).
6   Altman, F. and Zechner, G.: The pathology and pathogenesis of endolymphatic hydrops. New investigations. Arch. Ohr.- Nas.- KehlkHeilk. *192:* 1–19 (1968).
7   Shambaugh, G.E., jr.; Clemis, J.D., and Arenberg, I.K.: The endolymphatic sac and duct in Meniere's disease. Archs Otolar. *89:* 38–47 (1969).
8   Kohut, R.I. and Lindsay, J.R.: Pathologic changes in idiopathic labyrinthine hydrops. Correlations with previous findings. Acta oto-lar. *73:* 402–412 (1972).
9   Lindsay, J.R.: Effect of obliteration of the endolymphatic duct and sac in the monkey. Archs Otolar. *45:* 1–13 (1947).
10   Kimura, R.S. and Schuknecht, H.F.: Membranous hydrops in the inner ear of the guinea pig after obliteration of the endolymphatic sac. Pract. Oto-Rhino-Laryng. *27:* 343–354 (1065).

Robert A. Schindler, MD, The Saul and Ida Epstein Otoneurological Laboratory, Room 863-HSE, University of California, San Francisco, CA 94143 (USA)

Adv. Oto-Rhino-Laryng., vol. 25, pp. 134–137 (Karger, Basel 1979)

Caloric Nystagmus: ENG in Comparison with Observation by Frenzel's Glasses

P. Strauss and A. Meyer zum Gottesberge

ENT-Clinik, University of Düsseldorf, Düsseldorf

Material and Methods

In an experiment 30 test persons, between 20 and 30 years of age, underwent a caloric stimulation with water at 30°C for 30 sec. An electronystagmogram (ENG) was registered and simultaneously a second investigator observed the nystagmus by Frenzel's glasses and marked it on an additional canal of the ENG chart recorder [1, 2]. This simultaneous marking made it possible to decide for each nystagmus beat if this beat observed by Frenzel's glasses was really a defined nystagmus beat in the ENG.

The registration of an ENG and the simultaneous observation of the nystagmus by Frenzel's glasses result in the fact that the test conditions no longer correspond with the demand for standardization made by *Henriksson et al.* [3] in 1972: it is not registered in the darkness with eyes open, but the eyes are illuminated and their fixation is largely eliminated by Frenzel's glasses. The mental activity of test persons is comparatively high in solving arithmetical exercises. Compared with the registration in the darkness, the illumination of the eyes by Frenzel's glasses leads to a statistically based more intensive response of nystagmus concerning the parameters total duration, total number of beats and maximal frequency in the culmination interval [6]. In the course of our experiment one investigator records the ENG, a second investigator carries out the irrigation through a silicon catheter lying in the ear canal, and having finished this irrigation, he observes the nystagmus by Frenzel's glasses. At the same time he marks the observed nystagmus beats on the ENG recorder by pressing a button (fig. 1).

Results

The nystagmus registered by the ENG mostly starts when the calorization is not yet finished. The second investigator is still occupied with the irrigation so that he can neither observe the nystagmus by Frenzel's glasses nor mark it. The marking starts in the mean 23 sec later than the regis-

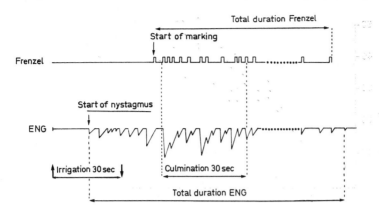

Fig. 1. Simultaneous registration of caloric nystagmus by means of ENG and marking by means of Frenzel's glasses.

tration of the nystagmus by the ENG. Using Frenzel's glasses the total duration, the total number of beats and the maximal frequency in the culmination interval are on a statistical base lower than registered by the ENG. Concerning the optimal reaction time, i.e. the period between the middle of the culmination interval and the end of the irrigation, there is, however, no essential difference. By the use of Frenzel's glasses there are nearly no nystagmus beats which do not correspond to a defined nystagmus beat in the ENG. Positive results being falsely registered only occur in the mean 1.7 times (the maximum is six times) when there are more than 200 total numbers of beats.

In comparison to ENG registration, the observation of the nystagmus by Frenzel's glasses results in a loss of information in quantity. The period of the nystagmus is, however, clearly reflected by Frenzel's glasses.

Discussion

How important is this loss of information, if the nystagmus is only observed by Frenzel's glasses? The loss of information is linear, it is small observing nystagmus beats of low frequency, if the frequency increases, it linearly increases with the frequency. This is true for the total number of beats as well as for the maximal frequency in the culmination interval (fig. 2). That means that the nystagmus observed by Frenzel's glasses reflects in all checked sections the intensity of the real defined nystagmus

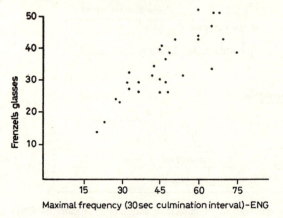

Fig. 2. Relationship between measuring in ENG and simultaneously observing Frenzel's glasses.

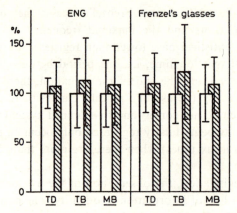

Fig. 3. Comparison between ENG and Frenzel's glasses, accuracy of registration. TD = Total duration; TB = total number of beats; MB = maximal number of beats (30 sec culm.). Irrigation of the right ear, 30 sec, 30 °C: open = relaxed; hatched = arithmetic. Standard deviation is shown; the underlining indicates statistically significantly different.

response. The amplitude of the nystagmus beats has only an insignificant influence on the identification of nystagmus beats by Frenzel's glasses.

The example of the change of mental activity from relaxation to an arithmetic task can be evidence that even by the simple observation of the nystagmus by Frenzel's glasses small changes of the intensity of reaction are registered on a statistical basis. The increase of mental activity leads by ENG registration in all parameters to a statistically based increase of nystagmus response. This comparatively small increase of the reaction can be equally precisely registered by the use of Frenzel's glasses only in all parameters concerning the frequency (fig. 3). Regarding the extent of the variation, there is no essential difference between the registration by ENG or Frenzel's glasses [5].

If the evaluation is limited to the frequency and if it is possible to neglect the velocity of the slow phase or the amplitude [4, 7], the simple observation of nystagmus by Frenzel's glasses and its marking on a time chart recorder is no less effective than an ENG for measuring the difference between the right and left labyrinth.

Summary

After caloric stimulation with water at 30°C for 30 sec an electronystagmogram (ENG) was registered. Simultaneously with the ENG the test person's nystagmus was observed by Frenzel's glasses. If the evaluation is limited to the frequency of the nystagmus and if it is possible to neglect the velocity of the slow phase, the simple observation through Frenzel's glasses and its plotting on a time chart recorder is no less effective than an ENG for measuring the difference between the right and left labyrinth.

References

1 Claussen, C.: Das Frequenzmaximum des kalorisch ausgelösten Nystagmus I als Kennlinienfunktion des geprüften Vestibularorgans. Acta oto-lar. 67: 639–645 (1969).

2 Claussen, C.: Das Frequenz-Nystagmogramm, eine einfache quantitative Nystagmus-dokumentation für die Praxis ohne Elektronystagmographie. HNO, Berl. 18: 216–220 (1970).

3 Henriksson, N.G.; Pfaltz, C.R.; Torok, N., and Rubin, W.: A synopsis of the vestibular system (Sandoz Monogr., Basel 1972).

4 Hinchcliffe, R.: Validity of measures of caloric test response. Acta oto-lar. 63: 69–73 (1967).

5 Strauss, P.; Schneider, J., und Kurzeja, A.: Ist die Auswertung des experimentellen kalorischen Nystagmus mit dem Elektronystagmographen genauer als mit der Frenzel Brille? HNO, Berl. 25: 154–155 (1977).

6 Strauss, P. and Meyer Zum Gottesberge, A.: The effect of mental activity on thermically induced nystagmus under changed test conditions. 6th Extaord. Meet. Bárány Soc., London 1977.

7 Torok, N.: The culmination phenomenon and frequency pattern of the thermic nystagmus. Acta oto-lar. 48: 530–533 (1957).

P. Strauss, MD, HNO-Klinik, Universität Düsseldorf, Moorenstrasse 5, D-4000 Düsseldorf 1 (FRG)

Adv. Oto-Rhino-Laryng., vol. 25, pp. 138–143 (Karger, Basel 1979)

Dynamic Evaluation of Human Vestibulo-Ocular Function Using White Noise Rotation Stimulus and Linear System Parameter Estimation Techniques

C. Wall III, F.O. Black and D.P. O'Leary

Eye and Ear Hospital, Department of Otolaryngology,
University of Pittsburgh School of Medicine, Pittsburgh, Pa.

Introduction

Although rotational stimulation has been used for sometime [*Barany,* 1907; *van Egmond et al.,* 1948] in attempts to infer vestibular function through the vestibular-ocular reflex (VOR), recent advances in signal processing and parameter estimation coupled with the inexorably decreasing costs of laboratory computers have brought the use of rotational testing nearer the realm of clinical reality. Normal data bases using harmonic testing [*Wolfe et al.,* 1978] and pseudorandom binary sequence (PRBS) white noise acceleration stimulation [*Wall et al.,* 1978a] are now being developed as a basis for comparison with data obtained from selected patients in a 'case study' approach. Characteristic patterns (for example, unilateral vs. bilateral peripheral lesions) are becoming evident by the examination of gain, phase and asymmetry measures. Results from both harmonic and PRBS stimulation have been roughly comparable.

In this report, we have used preliminary patient results from the PRBS rotational testing to suggest two potential schemes which might be used to classify VOR responses clinically. The first uses the calculated 'raw' gain and phase data together with a measure of asymmetry. The second scheme uses linear systems parameter fits in an attempt to reduce the number of data points while increasing the possibility of relating test results to physiological control system theory predictions.

Methods

The stimulus delivery system, slow phase velocity (SPV) reconstruction, gain and phase calculations are all identical to those used in the acquisition of normal data [*Wall et al.,* 1978a]. Briefly, a PRBS of rotational acceleration was selected to give a test bandwidth of 0.02–1.67 Hz. The response to this acceleration input is considered to be slow phase eye velocity. A VOR transfer function is calculated using cross-spectral techniques which also can yield a measure of the 'causality' of these system responses [*Bendat and Piersol,* 1971]. This measure, coherence, indicates whether the output of a system is directly and linearly related to the input or whether nonlinearities or noise contamination are present. Values for the coherence function lie in the range of one to zero. A value of one implies that the response or output of a system is related to the stimulus or input in a linear, noise-free way. If there are nonlinearities in the system, or if the response is contaminated with noise, then the coherence value will decrease. Coherence values cannot be used to distinguish between nonlinearities and noise.

The value of the *stimulus* velocity, averaged over time is zero. For normal subjects, the average value of the reconstruction SPV is also near zero ($-0.10 \pm 1.19°$ sec, *Wall et al.* [1978a]). By convention, a positive value indicates a reduced response to the right. The average value of the SPV for unilaterally labyrinthectomized patients was measured to use as an estimate of the asymmetry of the systems response. Pilot data for several patients typically showed a value of 3–8 ° sec using the PRBS stimulus previously described [*Wall et al.,* 1978b]. It is recognized that such an asymmetrical response is caused by the introduction of a nonlinear element into the VOR. In this case, although the linear systems descriptor does not completely characterize the response, it nevertheless serves as a first approximation of the nystagmus response and has clinical usefulness.

Linear systems parameters were also fit to the transfer function gain and phase data as previously described [*Peterka et al.,* 1978; *Wall et al.,* 1978a]. Two classes of abnormal responses were defined as: unilateral reduced response and bilateral reduced response. Data from patients having documented unilateral and bilateral defects were given caloric, postural and rotational testing in addition to a thorough physical examination.

Results

The results for patterns which occur in the 'raw' transfer function of pilot abnormal patients are reported in detail elsewhere [*Wall et al.,* 1978b]. In summary, the normal VOR transfer function appears to be linear for the test stimulus used since doubling or having the strength changes the transfer function calculations by less than 10%. We speculate that this small change is due primarily to improvement in the signal-to-noise ratio of the response as the stimulus strength is increased. There is no obvious saturation when the normal intensity stimulus was doubled in amplitude. Table I lists the coherence calculations for normal and pilot study abnormal PRBS white

Table I. Coherence values for normal and pilot abnormal white noise tests

	Frequency Hz	Coherence			
		Normal (n=30)		pilot unilateral lesion	pilot bilateral reduced response
		mean	SD		
1	0.02	0.96	0.06	0.92	0.82
2	0.05	0.85	0.09	0.69	0.18
3	0.11	0.62	0.20	0.64	0.09
4	0.23	0.38	0.21	0.47	0.003
5	0.46	0.17	0.11	0.30	0.01
6	0.93	0.09	0.05	0.08	0.05
7	1.67	0.02	0.02	0.03	0.03

Table II. Classification scheme for human VOR white noise rotation testing

Class of abnormality		Test parameter			
		gain	phase	coherence	mean SPV
I	Asymmetric Weak right Weak left	normal or slightly below normal	significantly above normal	slightly lower than normal	$<3°/sec$ $>-3°/sec$
II	Reduced bilateral	well below normal	not systematically distributed	much lower than normal	

noise tests. Note that the coherence for normal subjects progressively decreases with increasing frequency.

For the unilateral labyrinthectomy data, the coherence estimate (table I) for the first four frequency points are only slightly less than those calculated for normal subjects. The reduced coherences indicate the possibility of the introduction of a nonlinear element into the VOR causing an asymmetry in the case of a unilateral peripheral defect. For the patient with a reduced bilateral response the coherence values indicate that the response is abnormally insensitive to the stimulus, which is to be expected. This situation is also reflected in the gain calculations. Table II summarizes the results of the 'raw' transfer function classification scheme.

The linear system parameter fits characterize the transfer function in terms of a DC gain term, k, and a set of time constants, T_j [*Peterka et al.,* 1978]. Even though a third order fit has been made to the raw transfer

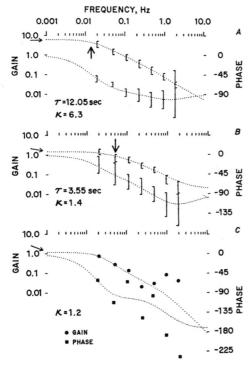

Fig. 1. A Linear systems fit to VOR transfer function from 30 normal subjects using white noise acceleration stimulation. A third order fit is shown. The two relevant parameters are the steady state gain, k, and the time constant, τ, corresponding to the corner frequency shown by the arrow. Plotted points are mean for 30 normal. Brackets are ±1 SD. Gain brackets point to left, phase brackets point to right. *B* Linear systems fit to pilot unilateral labyrinthectomy data. The corner frequency has increased to 0.045 Hz with a corresponding change in τ to 3.55 sec. Plotted points are estimated gain and phase. Brackets are 95% confidence intervals. *C* Linear systems fit to pilot bilaterally reduced VOR response. The steady state gain, k is 1.2. Confidence intervals are not plotted (see text).

function, the results from only one of the time constants will be presented here. This time constant relates to the so-called 'corner frequency' at which the gain curve fit is changing from a horizontal line to a downward sloping line. In the simplest case, the curve fit for the phase response is sloping downward and passes −45° at the corner frequency. For the group of 30 normal subjects, this point occurs at 0.013 Hz which corresponds to a 12.05 sec time constant shown in figure 1A. The value of the steady state gain for the ensemble of 30 normal subjects is 6.3.

The third order parameter fit for a patient having a unilateral laby-rinthectomy indicates that the above-mentioned corner frequency increases to 0.045 Hz with a resulting decrease in the time constant to 3.55 sec, as shown in figure 1B. This shift in the 'corner frequency' is more easily detected by comparing the phase points of figures 1A and B, recall that the gain and phase points are *simultaneously* fit using linear system parameters. It is important to note that the steady state gain of 1.4 for the unilateral case is also reduced as compared to normal.

The linear systems parameter fit for a patient showing reduced bi-lateral response is more difficult to interpret. Due to low coherence values (less than 0.25 except for the first point), the system response is not well related to the input or stimulus. This results in very wide confidence interl vals except for the first frequency point, at 0.02 Hz, the 95% confidence intervals were larger than the value of the gain estimate itself and are therefore not plotted. Nevertheless, the value of steady state gain which equals 1.23 in this case is greatly reduced when compared to that for nor-mal subjects.

Discussion

The 12.05 time constant has been obtained by the linear system para-meter fit of normal data, is in agreement with the 'long' time constant found from the analysis of the decaying SPV trace after an abrupt change in velocity such as those which occur in 'cupulometry' type vestibular stimuli [*van Egmond et al.,* 1948].

In cases where the coherence is suitably high, then a linear systems parameter fit in the frequency domain seems to be sensitive enough to detect changes in this time constant which are related to an abnormal vestibular function. We feel that if the parameter fit had been made to data obtained from harmonic rotational stimulation, the results would have been similar.

In cases where the coherence function is low, then a parameter fit seems to have less validity as a sorting approach. This is not an unexpected result. The 'raw' transfer function and coherence indicates in such a case that the response of the system is simply not related to the stimulus.

Although the parameter fit approach is more elegant, the comparison of 'raw' transfer function data offers an additional advantage. Namely, that confidence intervals can be placed around the data for each individual person, thereby facilitating comparisons with normal data. At this time, the accuracy of the linear systems parameter fit cannot be assigned a confidence interval.

Summary

White noise acceleration inputs were used to determine the human VOR transfer function both for normal subjects and for patients falling into two pilot categories: unilateral labyrinthectomy and reduced bilateral responses. The systematic patterns shown in the transfer function of the pilot abnormal categories as compared to the normal data suggests one method of classifying test results (table I). Frequency domain linear systems parameter fits were also made using the same data. The changes in these fit parameters, when pilot abnormal data is compared to normal data, suggests the use of the parameter fits themselves as a second classification scheme (fig. 1). The second scheme is not appropriate in cases where the response is unrelated to the stimulus.

References

Barany, R.: Weitere Untersuchungen über den vom Vestibularapparat des Ohres reflektorisch ausgelösten rhythmischen Nystagmus und seine Begleiterscheinungen. Mschr. Ohrenheilk. Lar.- Rhinol. *41:* 477 (1907).

Bendat, J.S. and Piersol, A.G.: Random data: analysis and measurement procedures (Wiley-Interscience, New York 1971).

Egmond, A.A.J. van; Groen, J.J., and Jongkees, L.B.W.: Turning test with small regulable stimuli: cupulometry. J. Laryng. *62:* 63–69 (1948).

Peterka, R.J.; O'Leary, D.P., and Tomko, D.L.: Linear system techniques for the evaluation of semicircular canal afferent responses using white noise rotational stimuli. Proc. VIth Extraordinary Meeting of Barany Society, 1978, pp. 10–17.

Wall, C., III; O'Leary, D.P., and Black, F.O.: Systems analysis of vestibulo-ocular system responses using white noise rotational stimuli. Proc. VIth Extraordinary Meeting of Barany Society, 1978a pp. 157–164.

Wall, C., III; Black, F.O., and O'Leary, D.P.: Clinical use of pseudorandom binary sequence white noise in assessment of human vestibulo-ocular reflex. Ann. Otol. Rhinol. Lar. (to be published, 1978b).

Wolfe, J.W.; Engelken, E.J., and Kos, C.M.: Low-frequency harmonic acceleration as a test of labyrinthine function: basic methods and illustrative cases. Otolaryng. *86:* ORL-130 (1978).

C. Wall III, PhD, Eye and Ear Hospital, Department of Otolaryngology, University of Pittsburgh School of Medicine, Pittsburgh, PA 15213 (USA)

Adv. Oto-Rhino-Laryng., vol. 25, pp. 144–148 (Karger, Basel 1979)

Characteristics of Body Sway in Patients with Peripheral Vestibular Disorders

K. Taguchi

Department of Otolaryngology (Director: Prof. *T. Suzuki*),
Faculty of Medicine, Shinshu University, Matsumoto

Introduction

The eye movements and the nystagmus observed in the patients with peripheral vestibular disorders have been reported by many authors, however, the body sway of the same patient has been given little attention. The righting reflex, characterized by Romberg's test, has been an important tool in neurological diagnosis. There seem to be some characteristics of body sway particular to the standing human suffering from vertigo. The righting reflex is usually disturbed to some extent in vertiginous patients during standing with the eyes closed, especially in patients suffering from vestibular disorders. The body's center of gravity (CG) moves regularly or irregularly and the measurement of CG movement nearly represents the objective righting reflex.

The present study deals with the signs observed in the CG movement of the patients with peripheral vestibular disorders.

Methods and Material

The static sensonograph applying strain gauge technique (Sanei Co. Tokyo, Japan) was used to obtain, from a subject standing on the platform of the apparatus, a continuous record of CG movement in the horizontal plane. The output, in terms of voltage, from the sensonograph is connected to a plotting unit. The information obtained was at the same time supplied to a data recorder, which separately stored the data of the lateral and anteroposterior CG movement on the tape. The recorded data on the tape were fed into a digital computer for calculating the length of locus and the time course in the averaged position of CG, and analyzing the frequency spectrum of CG movement.

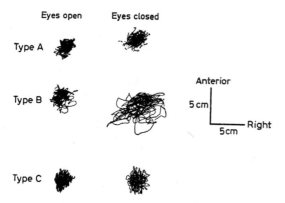

Fig. 1. Locus patterns of the patients with peripheral vestibular disorders. They were classified into three types according to the figures traced by the body's center of gravity during 1 min standing with the eyes closed.

The experiments were conducted on 30 patients with peripheral vestibular disorders. Each subject was placed on the platform of the sensonograph with feet together and asked to look straight ahead. Recordings were made with the eyes open and with the eyes closed. Each set of recordings was repeated three times in order to verify the reliability of the examination.

Results

The Patterns of Locus Traced by CG Movement during Normal Standing. The Locus was plotted on graphic paper by an XY recorder. Calibrations were made to let 1 cm in the CG displacement be replaced by 1 cm of the traced locus on the graphic paper of the XY recorder after making corrections depending on the body weight and the height of subjects at every measurement.

The patterns obtained from the normal subject showed a centripetal or concentric configuration, while the patients with peripheral vestibular disorders represented various patterns of locus which became significantly larger by eye-closing. In the subjects with peripheral vestibular disorders three types of locus patterns were classified according to the figures traced during standing with the eye closed (fig. 1, table I). The first type resembled closely that of normal subjects except for the area occupied by the locus and it was designated Type A. The second type was Type B in which the lateral component of locus exceeded the anteroposterior component in the

Table I. Types of the locus patterns traced by the center of gravity

	Number of subjects (cases)	
	with nystagmus	without nystagmus
Type A	2	12
Type B	9	1
Type C	1	5
Total	12	18

moving range of CG. Type C had the characteristic pattern in which the antero-posterior component exceeded the lateral component in the length of locus.

The Total Length of Locus Traced by CG during Standing. In normal subjects the total length of locus traced by CG during 1 min standing was 53.2 ± 17.1 cm with the eyes open and 78.6 ± 30.2 cm with the eyes closed. In the subjects with peripheral vestibular disorders the length was 60.2 ± 22.8 cm with the eyes open and 96.7 ± 49.6 cm with the eyes closed. A certain relationship between the types of the locus pattern and the total length of locus was proved. In the test with the eyes open the subject group with Type B showed the minimal value of locus length and the group with Type C had the maximal value, while in the tests with the eyes closed the group with Type B showed the maximal and the group with Type C had the minimal value.

The Time Course in the Averaged Position of CG. The averaged position of CG was calculated every 10 sec and figured as the sequential punctual coordinate. The patients with the spontaneous nystagmus showed a characteristic time course of CG position, that is, the CG shift toward the direction of the slow phase of the nystagmus. However, no tendency was obtained from the patients with fine or no nystagmus.

The Frequency Spectra of the CG Movement. Frequency spectra of the CG movement were calculated using a Fourier technique. A preliminary study revealed that the main frequency related to CG movement was observed below 3 Hz, and therefore the frequency analysis of the CG movement done within the range of 1/60 to 3 Hz. The frequency analysis of the CG movement of the patients with peripheral vestibular disorders resulted

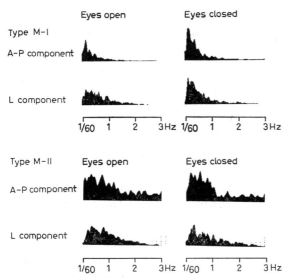

Fig. 2. Frequency spectra of the patients with Meniere's disease. Two types (Type M-I and Type M-II) were characteristic of Meniere's disease.

in some diversity of the data. However, the frequency spectra of the patients with Meniere's disease were classified into two types (fig. 2).

Discussion

Several authors reported the characteristics of the body sway in the patients with peripheral vestibular disorders. *Kapteyn and de Wit* [1972] reported that patients suffering from Meniere's disease showed irregular locus with a low frequency of about 0.2 Hz. *Dichgans et al.* [1976] mentioned that the body sway of the patients with vestibular lesions was very heterogenous and the diversity of the data in the patients might reflect the high ability for a central compensation.

There has been few data on the normal range of the length of locus traced by CG. In the present study there was no significant difference between the length of normal subjects and the patients with vestibular disorders with the eyes open, while there was a statistically significant difference when the eyes were closed. This result would indicate a characteristic of the body sway in the vestibular disorders and probably means the presence of the visual compensation during standing with the eyes open.

The time course of CG position measured every 10 sec in normal subjects was restricted. *Kapteyn and de Wit* [1972] showed the more excentric locus of the abnormal cases. *Taguchi et al.* [1977] reported that 14 of 41 patients with vestibular disorders showed abnormal time course when the eyes were open and 21 subjects showed abnormal value with the eyes closed.

The frequency spectrum obtained from CG movement indicates whether the subject's body maintains a regular sway and at what frequency the body moves. *Tokita et al.* [1970] and *Matsuoka* [1977] reported that the patients with peripheral vestibular disorders moved at the frequency of 0.2 Hz. On the contrary, *Dichgans et al.* [1976] stated that there was no characteristic frequency in the vestibular lesions. The present study showed that there was a close relationship between the frequency spectra and Meniere's disease.

Summary

Measuring the movement of the body's center of gravity during standing with the eyes open and with the eyes closed, proved to be a useful test in vestibular investigation. 30 patients with peripheral vestibular disorders were tested using a static sensonograph and a digital computer. Three types of locus patterns, the lateral deviation of the averaged position and two types of frequency spectral patterns obtained from the movement of the center of gravity were the characteristics of the body sway in the patients with peripheral vestibular disorders.

References

Dichgans, J.; Mauritz, K.-H.; Allum, J.-H.-J., and Brandt, T.: Postural sway in normals and atactic patients: analysis of the stabilizing and destabilizing effects of vision. Agressologie *17:* 15–24 (1976).
Kapteyn, T.S. and de Wit, G.: Posturography as an auxiliary in vestibular investigation. Acta oto-lar. *73:* 104–111 (1972).
Matsuoka, T.: Quantitative analysis of the body sway while standing. Pract. Otol., Kyoto *70:* 1191–1280 (1977).
Taguchi, K.; Iijima, M., and Takizawa, M.: Spectral analysis of the movement of the body's center of gravity. Frequency spectrum and averaged divisional frequency. Pract. Otol., Kyoto *70:* 825–831 (1977).
Tokita, T.; Miyata, H.; Fujita, H.; Nagata, T.; Kobayashi, T.; Kato, K.; Kato, Y.; Taguchi, T.; Shima, R.; Suzuki, T., and Hibi, H.: Correlation analysis of body-sways in standing posture. Pract. Otol., Kyoto *63:* 363–387 (1970).

K. Taguchi, MD, Department of Otolaryngology, Faculty of Medicine,
Shinshu University, 1-1 Asahi 1-Chomo, Matsumoto (Japan)

Adv. Oto-Rhino-Laryng., vol. 25, pp. 149–155 (Karger, Basel 1979)

Some Critical Remarks on the Interpretation of Vestibular Test Results

Marcel E. Norré

Vestibular Department, Akademisch Ziekenhuis, University of Leuven, Leuven

In the scope of the diagnosis of peripheral lesions, functional value of the vestibular system is the most important datum to be obtained from the examination. Whereas qualitative disturbances, such as failure of fixation suppression (FFS), ocular dissociation, hyperreflexia, dysrhythmias, opto-motor anomalies, are typical features of central disturbance; in peripheral diseases, it is a fundamental question whether a normal function or a partial or complete loss of function – mostly of one system – is present. Here *asymmetrical peripheral function* is the cause of the imbalance and *source of the vertigo.* About this peripheral imbalance we are informed by the caloric tests. Besides, it is of utmost importance to evaluate also the *global functioning of the system,* whatever the peripheral function may be. This evaluation is realized by the rotation tests [4, 6].

An absolute evaluation of function clearly seems of less importance, because of the widespread range of normal values. So we consider, with *Jongkees* [2], *relative measurement* as fundamental for the evaluation of the peripheral function. In this way it is indicated whether or not both systems act in equilibrium, i.e. whether they have nearly the same input. This is the basic evaluation of the peripheral function and the side difference, thus obtained, we call *'peripheral imbalance'.* In the same way, central regulation mechanisms are expressed by the equilibrated or dysequilibrated reaction resulting from rotation tests. Here too, the relative balance state between both nystagmus directions informs us about this *'central balance'.* We compute it in the same relative way [4–6].

However, we observe that the *values of stimulation,* used in all these tests, may be *very different* from one author to the other. This is the case not only for caloric tests, but more strikingly for rotation tests. The latter, moreover, may be performed according to different types of stimulation: the acceleration test, the postrotatory reaction, the pendular or other alternating tests.

The results of these tests should inform us about this functional value of the vestibular system we mentioned above. When such a test shows us some functional relationship between the two systems in the caloric tests, or between the two nystagmus directions in both caloric and rotation tests, we are inclined to take this datum, *expressing the functional capacity of the system in an absolute manner*. When one system is reacting to the stimulus we applied at a lower level than the other one, we call this system hyporeflective, hypoexcitable (or canal paresis according to *Hallpike*). We consider this to be a quality inherent to this examined system, i.e. that we admit implicitly that this system will always react in this inferior way, no matter the intensity of the stimulus which will be applied. The same holds true for rotation tests, when we conclude whether or not compensation is realized, according to the degree of balance between both nystagmus directions, obtained by application of only one stimulus intensity or type.

However, when we apply *more than one intensity or type of stimulation*, we have to admit that such an assumption, in no way, holds true for all the cases. Summarizing our experience [4, 6] concerning the results of the application of stimulations of more than one intensity, our cases can be divided in two groups: the cases in which we effectively find the same functional relationship for every intensity applied, and the group in which the *result is dependent on the intensity* and, for rotation tests, *even on the type of the stimulus*. Other authors [1, 3, 7, 8] too have found such discordances, interpreting them mostly in the scope of the notions of recruitment and decruitment. We could gather extensive experience [4, 6] concerning this problem, as we could examine a series of patients (n = 474) on which we applied a combined scheme of rotation tests, and also a series of cases (n = 162) stimulated calorically at 20 °C after the performing of the 'classical' stimulation level of *Hallpike* at 30/44 °C.

Caloric Results

Concerning the caloric test results, we could observe following data:

The cases were first examined at 30/44 °C and the results were computed in the classical way, based on the maximal slow phase velocity at the culmination point. Here we applied the formula of *Jongkees:*

Table I. Comparison of the caloric results obtained by the caloric stimulations at 30/44 °C and 20 °C

Results at 20 °C	Caloric asymmetry 30/44° (n = 109)	Caloric symmetry 30/44° (n = 53)
Same relation	51 (46.78 %)	41 (77.35 %)
=	24	
+	13	
−	14	
Different	58 (53.12 %)	
20 °C symmetry	39	
20 °C inversed	19	
20 °C asymmetry		12 (22.64 %)

$$\frac{R-L}{R+L} \times 100.$$

A difference of 20 % and more was accepted as significant and such a reaction was considered as an *imbalance*. The same computing was executed for the results of the 20 °C stimulation.

Comparing the results of the 30/44 °C and of the 20 °C stimulation, we can observe that some cases have concordant results, others show a discordant one. Table I shows our results in a series of 162 cases. We point out that only 92 (56.79 %) show a same relationship between the two systems (either symmetry or asymmetry in the same sense) for both stimulation levels, 30/44 °C and 20 °C. On the other hand, we have 70 cases which show different balance states at 20 °C. So the imbalance at 30/44 °C disappeared at 20 °C in 39 cases; this event can be considered as a recruitment phenomenon [1]. In 19 cases 20 °C stimulation shows an inversed relationship: the formerly hypofunctional side becomes dominant. On the contrary, 12 cases among 53 with symmetrical reaction at 30/44 °C show asymmetry at 20 °C. This clearly proves that in a nonnegligible number of cases, the finding of unilateral hypofunction is related to stimulus intensity. Indeed in 70 cases (43.20 %) it was intensity dependent.

Rotatory Results

As rotation tests we used three types:
(a) The *acceleratory* stimulation: i.e., application of a continuous fixed acceleration during

Table II. Number of cases showing an inbalance in each of the three stimulation levels of the acceleratory and postrotatory reaction: the same for the pendular test according to three modes of evaluation; the number of cases showing a labile and those showing a stable reaction pattern in the three rotatory stimulation types

Imbalances	Stimulation level					
	I		II		III	
	n	%	n	%	n	%
Acceleratory	235	49.57	207	43.67	162	34.57
Postrotatory	187	39.45	142	30.01	100	21.09
	Frequency		Velocity		Frequency + velocity	
Pendular	126	26.58	108	22.78	153	32.27
	Reaction patterns					
	Labile		Stable		Insufficient reaction	
Acceleratory	313	66.03	126	26.58	35	7.80
Postrotatory	269	56.75	204	43.03	1	7.00
Pendular (n = 229)	56	24.45	166	72.48	7	3.05

30 sec. We used 1, 2, 4°/sec^2, stimulation levels resp. I, II, III. (b) The *postrotatory reaction:* realized by a stop in 1 sec from constant rotation during 2 min at 30° and 60°/sec and in $1^1/_3$ sec from 120°/sec, stimulation levels resp. I, II, III. (c) A *sinusoidal pendular* rotation type.

Table II shows the number of cases presenting rotatory imbalance at acceleratory, postrotatory and pendular tests. This number decreases from level I to III, and there is a difference between both types of stimulation. Moreover, it has to be emphasized that this does not mean gradation in imbalance, but that imbalance in III does not imply necessarily the presence of imbalance in II and I; the presence of the imbalances being independently spread over the three levels. As a result of this spread, we could define some specific *reaction patterns.*

An imbalance in I, clearly diminished or absent in II and III, is called a *recruitment pattern*. The inverse relation means a *decruitment pattern,* whereas we call it a *V pattern*

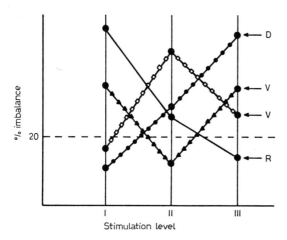

Fig. 1. Reaction patterns. R (recruitment): a significant imbalance (>20%) in level I disappears in level III. D (decruitment) has the inversed evolution. V (variable) gives two types.

when variable distribution is present with only imbalance in II, or in I and III (cfr scheme of figure 1.) These patterns are called 'labile' patterns in contradistinction with those showing an equal state of balance or imbalance in the three levels (stable patterns).

We let aside the discussion of these patterns with regard to the notions of recruitment and decruitment. In the scope of our present discussion, we would like to point out that a case showing one of the mentioned patterns can be considered as *balanced or imbalanced, according to the level of stimulation which is taken into consideration.* Table II shows the sum of the cases showing such patterns, for the three stimulation types.

We would like to emphasize that a difference is to be noted, not only according to stimulation intensity, but also according to *stimulation type.* This holds for the absolute number of cases showing imbalance as well as for the number presenting the described reaction patterns. Once more it appears that the presence of imbalance – or some reaction pattern – in one stimulation type does not imply the presence of the same reaction type in the other one. We notice that, when no imbalance is shown in the post-rotatory reactions (n = 184), in 116 among them there is a pattern of imbalance in the acceleration test; and inversely, when the acceleratory tests are in balance (n = 98), 43 show imbalance in one or more of the post-rotation levels.

Conclusions

These data amply confirm our thesis: *the results of the tests are to be taken in a relative way and the functional evaluation is not an absolute feature of the functional capacity of the examined system,* as in nearly half of the cases intensity and/or type dependence is to be taken into account.

This relativation of results is an important datum, when we wish to compare results of various investigators, performing tests according to different schemes. Our findings argue in favor of some *standardization* of, at least, the basic evaluation tests.

Especially for the rotation tests, it seems very interesting *to apply more than one type or intensity* of stimulus in order to evaluate the central regulation function, particularly for those cases showing peripheral imbalance and when we wish to have some precise information about the state of central compensation [5]. Indeed, we observe that in some cases, this compensation seems to be *stable,* being the same, i.e. of the same degree, no means which is the 'loading', in others it seems to be *labile,* dependent on type or intensity of the 'loading'. These statements constituted the basis and starting point of the development of a special treatment: the 'vestibular habituation training' [6].

Summary

In the scope of the evaluation of vestibular function, the attention is drawn to the fact that results of tests are to be considered in a relative way. They do not express the absolute functional capacity, but in half of the cases it can be shown that the functional state is intensity dependent. This can be observed in caloric tests as well as in rotation tests. In these latter even the type of stimulation may give a different result. The experiences obtained in a number of cases by both stimulation types confirm this assessment that the functional result is always to be considered in this relative way. This implies some reserves as to the comparability of results of various authors, using different stimulation schemes. On the other hand, and this especially in rotation tests, application of more stimulation intensities allows to separate cases with stable from those with labile results.

References

1   Gramowski, K.H.: Über die sogenannte vestibuläre Rekruitment. Z. Lar. Rhinol. Otol. *51:* 601–605 (1972).

2   Jongkees, L.B.W.: The caloric test and its value in the evaluation of the patient with vertigo. Otolar. Clins N. Am. *6:* 73–93 (1973).

3   Litton, W.B. and MacCabe, B.F.: Thermal vestibulometry; in Graham, Sensori-neural hearing processes and disorders, pp. 263–268 (Little, Brown, Boston 1967).

4   Norré, M.E.: ENG-bevindingen bij eenzijdig vestibulair functieverlies; thesis University of Leuven (1977).

5   Norré, M.E.: The importance of rotatory proofs. Acta oto-rhino-lar. belg. *31:* 89–98 (1977).

6   Norré, M.E.: The unilateral vestibular hypofunction. Acta oto-rhino-lar. belg. *32:* 421–668 (1978).

7   Torok, N.: Differential caloric stimulations in vestibular diagnosis. Archs Otolar. *90:* 52–56 (1969).

8   Reker, U.; Rudert, H. und Heimke, U.: Untersuchungen zum vestibulären Rekruitment. Lar. Rhinol. Otol. *54:* 248–256 (1975).

M.E. Norré, MD, PhD, Head of the Vestibular Department,
Akademisch Ziekenhuis, University of Leuven, Leuven (Belgium)

Adv. Oto-Rhino-Laryng., vol. 25, pp. 156–160 (Karger, Basel 1979)

Peripheral Vestibular Disorder of Cervical Origin

Jiro Hozawa

Department of Otolaryngology, Hirosaki University School of Medicine, Hirosaki

Introduction

When transient episodes of vertigo are induced by movement of the head and neck, the cervicovestibular syndrome may be suspected. In such cases, the following findings can often be made: (1) peripheral or central vestibular disorders; (2) spondylosis deformans (revealed by X-ray photography); (3) abnormality of the vertebral artery (revealed by angiography).

Since 1963, the author has treated patients suffering from the cervicovestibular syndrome by performing perivascular sympathectomy in the proximal part of the vertebral artery. This operation was very effective in cases of peripheral vestibular disorder. On the basis of the operational results, the provoking mechanism of peripheral vestibular disorder in the cervicovestibular syndrome is discussed.

Operative procedure

Under general anesthesia, the patient was placed in the supine position and the head was extended and rotated to the opposite side. An anterior approach was found to be preferable. The dissection of the subclavian triangle was carried out by making a 5-cm, slightly curved incision in the fascia of the neck (fig. 1a). The sternocleidomastoid muscle was exposed (fig. 1b) and divided (fig. 1c) or retracted towards the larynx; the phrenic nerve could be seen on the scalenus muscle (fig. 1d). The scalenus muscle was then retracted peripherally to expose the vertebral artery. This artery arises from the upper and posterior portion of the subclavian artery (fig. 1e). The adventitious coat of the vertebral artery was then stripped from its origin to its entrance into the foramina in the transverse process of the sixth cervical vertebra. The side to be operated on was decided by audiometric findings, the positioning test and vertebral angiography.

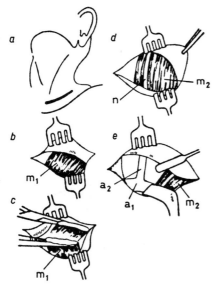

Fig. 1. Method of 'perivascular sympathectomy'. *a–e* Operation procedure.

Diagnosis of Peripheral Type of Cervicovestibular Syndrome

Positioning Test. Rotatory nystagmus can be provoked by the positioning test, and so-called *Gegenläuufigkeit* [*Stenger*, 1955] is often observed. When the test is repeated, fatigue due to nystagmus [*Lindsay*, 1951] can be observed.

Self-Recording Cupulometry. Hozawa and Sasaki [1968] devised a new rotation test for the purpose of differential diagnosis between peripheral vestibular disorder and central disorder. The testing method is as follows. Sitting in an electrically driven, revolving chair, the patient bends the head forward at an angle of 30°. During the test, the eye movements are recorded by ENG and can be observed through an infrared television camera at the same time. Prior to the test, the rate of angular acceleration is adjusted, and then the revolving chair is accelerated or decelerated. During the rotation of this chair, the latency time of nystagmus induced by acceleration or deceleration can be automatically recorded by referring to the tachograph on the chair. If there is a difference between the responses of the two labyrinths, the tachograph shows divergence from the baseline. This test is performed mainly to detect the presence or absence of this divergence phenomenon at

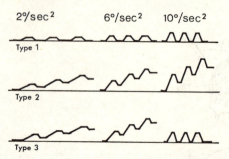

Fig. 2. Classification of the self-recording cupulogram. Type I: the effects of acceleration and deceleration are identical. The final point (L) is always on the baseline. This type is normal. Type II: the self-recording cupulogram always shows a divergence from the baseline. This type is caused by a directional preponderance (DP). Type III: the self-recording cupulogram showing the divergence with a weaker stimulation ($2°/sec^2$) reverts to the baseline in accordance with the increase of stimulation ($6°$ or $10°/sec^2$). This type is found exclusively in cases of peripheral lesion, but not of central lesion.

each stimulation of 2, 6 and $10°/sec^2$. The authors have named this test 'self-recording cupulometry' and the tachograph of the revolving chair 'the self-recording cupulogram'. The self-recording cupulogram can be classified in three types (fig. 2). Type I is normal and the divergence phenomenon is not observed at any degree of stimulation. In type II, divergence is always found. This originates from directional preponderance. Type III shows the divergence phenomenon due to a weaker stimulation. But the self-recording cupulogram reverts to the baseline in accordance with the increse of stimulation, and the divergence cannot be found. The authors have called this 'the reversion phenomenon'. This reversion phenomenon is similar in appearance to auditory recruitment and is a peculiar sign of peripheral vestibular disorder.

Results of Operation

In the 13 years from 1966 to 1978, 48 cases of the peripheral type of cervicovestibular syndrome have been treated by perivascular sympathectomy. The results are as follows:

	Improvement	Recurrence
Unilateral operation (48 cases)	42	6
Bilateral operation (6 cases)	6	0

The operation was performed first on the severely affected side. 42 patients could be completely cured of episodes of vertigo by unilateral operation, but the other 6 cases required bilateral operations to prevent such episodes.

During the operation, nystagmus was often provoked by stimulation around the proximal vertebral artery. The direction of the nystagmus corresponded closely to that of the positioning nystagmus prior to the operation. On the other hand, sympathetic nerve fibers could be found in the areolar tissues surrounding the artery by postoperative histopathologic examination.

Discussion

From the results obtained, it was thought that the occurrence of the cervicovestibular syndrome was closely connected with the vasomotor reflex. When the head was rotated or the neck was extended, two causal factors were thought to induce the abnormal vasomotor reflex. The first was mechanical compression of the vertebral artery by skeletal or muscular structures. These mechanical pressures on the vertebral artery were thought to stimulate the perivascular, sympathetic nerve plexus and to induce vasoconstriction. During the operation, nystagmus similar to positioning nystagmus could be provoked by electrically stimulating the adventitious coat of the vertebral artery. The second cause of the vasomotor reflex was a disturbance of the flow in the vertebral artery. When a 1% solution of methylene blue was injected into the dog's unilateral vertebral artery, it was observable in the ipsilateral branch of the basilar artery, as in McDonald's observation. The transient ischemia resulting in the ipsilateral branch of the basilar arter would provoke vasoconstriction. Even though the operation was limited to the perivascular sympathectomy, without correcting the abnormal vessel or removing the cervical spondylotic spurs, the patients were relieved from episodes of vertigo. The effects of this operation are thought to be due to the blocking not of the afferent but of the efferent pathway for the vasomotor reflex.

Conclusion

48 cases of peripheral vestibular disorder of cervical origin were treated by perivascular sympathectomy in the proximal part of the vertebral artery.

It was thought that the effectiveness of this operation was due to the blocking of the efferent impulses which caused vasoconstriction.

Summary

The provoking mechanism of peripheral vestibular disorder in the cervicovestibular syndrome is discussed on the basis of the results of perivascular sympathectomy of the vertebral artery. The peripheral type of this syndrome can be differentiated from the central type in that it shows fatigue due to positioning nystagmus and the reversion phenomenon in the self-recording cupulogram. 42 cases of the peripheral type could be completely cured of episodes of vertigo by the unilateral operation, but the other 6 cases required bilateral operations to prevent such episodes.

References

Field, W.: Effects of vascular disorders on the vestibular system: in Fields, neurological aspects of auditory and vestibular disorders. (Thomas, Springfield 1964).

Hozawa, J. and Sasaki, Y.: Self-recording cupulometry and its clinical value. Otol. Fukuoka *14:* suppl. 1, pp. 83–88 (1968).

McDonald, D.A. and Potter, J.M.: Distribution of blood to the brain. J. Physiol. *114:* 353–371 (1951).

Lindsay, J.R.: Postural vertigo and positional nystagmus. Ann. Otol. *60:* 1134–1149 (1951).

Stenger, H.H.: Über Lagerungsnystagmus unter besonderer Berücksichtigung des gegenläufigen transitorischen Provokationsnystagmus bei Lagewechsel in der Sagitalebene. Arch. Ohr.- Nas.- u. Kehlk. Heilk. *168:* 220–268 (1955).

J. Hozawa, MD, Department of Otolaryngology, Hirosaki University School of Medicine, Hirosaki (Japan)

Adv. Oto-Rhino-Laryng., vol. 25, pp. 161–166 (Karger, Basel 1979)

The Mechanism of
Benign Paroxysmal Positional Nystagmus

R.W. Baloh, S. Sakala and V. Honrubia

Reed Neurological Research Center, Department of Neurology and Department of Surgery/Division of Head and Neck (Otolaryngology), UCLA School of Medicine, Los Angeles, Calif.

Introduction

The pathophysiology and clinical significance of benign paroxysmal positional nystagmus (BPPN) have been subjects of continuous controversy. It is difficult for one to compare publications on so-called 'typical' BPPN since most reports do not include recordings of the nystagmus. Whether the direction of BPPN is always the same and whether paroxysmal positional nystagmus of central origin differs in direction is not established. BPPN is usually described as rotatory with the upper pole of the eye beating toward the undermost ear [1]. The consistency of this pattern and the amplitude of the actual horizontal and vertical components in each eye have not, to our knowledge, been reported. If, as *Schuknecht* [2] suggests, BPPN originates from the posterior canal of the undermost ear, it should have similar horizontal and vertical components in each patient, i.e., those predicted by the known anatomical connections between the posterior canal and the extra-ocular muscles. Furthermore, the slow component velocity profile obtained from recordings of BPPN should be helpful for understanding the dynamics of the abnormal posterior canal cupula. With these practical and theoretical considerations in mind we have studied electro-oculographic (EOG) recordings of BPPN from 8 patients.

Case Material and Methods

Bilateral monocular horizontal and vertical eye movements were recorded using EOG in 8 patients with BPPN. Details of the recording system are reported elsewhere [3]. The nystagmus was induced by a rapid change from the sitting to the head-hanging right and head-hanging left positions (as described by *Dix and Hallpike* [1]). The patient's eyes were opened behind Frenzel glasses in a darkened room. The duration of the standard position change was approximately 2 sec. The effects of slower and more rapid positional changes were also studied.

Each patient reported a typical history of brief episodes of vertigo induced by position change and each demonstrated paroxysmal positional nystagmus that fatigued on repeated positioning. In 7 patients BPPN occurred in only one head-hanging position while in one it occurred in both. In the latter patient the nystagmus was prominent in only one position and its direction was the same in both positions. The clinical diagnoses were as follows: posttraumatic, 2, vestibulopathy of unknown cause (BPPN and a vestibular paresis [3] on caloric testing), 2, and idiopathic (isolated), 4.

Results

The direction and amplitude of the horizontal and vertical components of BPPN were consistent. In all 8 cases the eye ipsilateral to the down ear had the largest horizontal component and its fast phase direction was away from the undermost ear. The direction of the fast phase of the horizontal component in the contralateral eye varied. In 6 of 8 patients the contralateral eye beat in the opposite direction of the ipsilateral eye, in one patient both eyes beat in the same direction and in the other there was no discernible horizontal component in the contralateral eye. The vertical component was always upbeat in both eyes but the eye contralateral to the undermost ear had a larger vertical amplitude. 4 of 8 patients demonstrated a low velocity rotatory nystagmus in the opposite direction after the paroxysmal positional nystagmus disappeared.

Figure 1 illustrates a composite slow component velocity (SCV) profile of BPPN in the head-hanging right position. The peak SCV of the vertical and horizontal vectors is different in each eye. The eye ipsilateral to the undermost ear reaches the highest peak SCV in the horizontal plane while the contralateral eye has the highest peak SCV in the vertical plane. The maximum SCV in the vertical plane was on average 3 times that of the horizontal plane. The time constant of the SCV rise for the vertical component varied from 1.5 to 4 sec while that of the SCV fall varied from 5 to 12 sec.

The peak SCV in both the horizontal and vertical planes was positively correlated with the speed of the positioning maneuver. If the second positioning was more rapid than the first the peak SCV was increased despite the expected fatigue. If the patient was slowly positioned from sitting to head-hanging over a 20-sec period, paroxysmal positional nystagmus was not in-

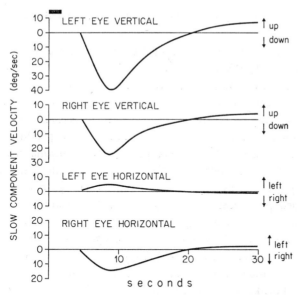

Fig. 1. Typical slow component velocity profile of benign paroxysmal positional nystagmus in the head-hanging right position. Arrows indicate the direction of the slow components. Solid bar indicates duration of positioning maneuver.

duced. By contrast the latency from the end of positioning to the onset of paroxysmal positional nystagmus decreased as speed of positioning increased.

Discussion

The direction of the horizontal and vertical vectors of BPPN are consistent with a burst of excitatory activity originating in the posterior canal of the undermost ear. Since the posterior canal has excitatory connections to the ipsilateral superior oblique and the contralateral inferior rectus [4] the slow components are directed downward and the fast components upward in both eyes. A larger horizontal component in the ipsilateral eye and a larger vertical component in the contralateral eye occur because of the different angle of insertion of the oblique and rectus muscles. The amplitude of the horizontal component in each eye also depends on the position of the eyes in the orbit when the BPPN begins. Disconjugate movements similar to those observed with BPPN have been produced in animals after selective stimulation of the ampullary nerve from a single posterior canal [5].

The observation that the fast phase of BPPN is directed upward is useful for distinguishing BPPN from other varieties of paroxysmal positional nystagmus. We have found that paroxysmal positional nystagmus caused by documented central nervous system lesions is usually downbeat (in the standard head-hanging position). The studies of *Fernandez* and co-workers [6–8] are often cited as evidence that BPPN can be produced by central lesions. These investigators produced paroxysmal positional nystagmus by ablating the posterior vermis of the cerebellum of the cat. They concluded that the positional nystagmus was a typical 'benign paroxysmal type' since it fatigued on repeated positioning and disappeared in a few days or weeks. Inspection of the nystagmus recordings [8], however, reveals important differences from BPPN as outlined in this report. The paroxysmal nystagmus induced by cerebellar lesions was always downbeat and its duration varied from 30 to 180 sec. The nystagmus intensity fluctuated, often demonstrating several peaks before slowly disappearing. Minimal horizontal components were observed and there was no mention of dissociation between the two eyes.

One can speculate about the mechanism of BPPN based on the SCV profile shown in the figure. Clearly the speed of the positioning maneuver is a key factor in determining the magnitude of induced nystagmus. BPPN does not occur if the head-hanging position is reached slowly. Therefore, the force of gravity alone is not the stimulus that induces BPPN. With the initial acceleration backward and to the side there is an ampullofugal displacement of the cupulae of the ipsilateral posterior canal and the contralateral anterior canal. With deceleration to the head-hanging position the cupulae return and then deviate slightly in the ampullopetal direction before finally returning to the mid-position. Assuming the anterior canal is functioning normally a brief positioning nystagmus occurs first beating upward (from ampullofugal displacement) and then downward (from ampullopetal displacement). As in normal subjects this positioning nystagmus is finished within a few seconds after the head-hanging position is reached.

The burst of BPPN could represent a delayed positioning nystagmus from the ipsilateral posterior canal. Its cupula does not respond instantaneously because of an attached external mass (such as Schuknecht's otolithic deposits [2]) or because of degenerative changes. Normally the short time constant of the cupula is about 5 msec, but because of central nervous system integration the peak slow component velocity after an impulse of acceleration does not occur until after a delay of about 0.5–1 sec [9]. The long latency represents the time required to 'charge' the central integrator. The delayed and temporally dispersed signal generated by the abnormal posterior canal would result in even longer latencies probably in the range of 5–10 sec. These prolonged latencies in ocular response are analogous to those seen after stimulation of the otolith organs by impulses of linear acceleration [10]. In other words, the cupula of the posterior semicircular canal is altered in such a way that its mechanical properties approach those of the otoliths. This hypothesis can be tested by observing the response to an impulse of acceleration in the plane of the damaged posterior canal. Two nystagmus responses should occur, one from stimulation of the normal anterior canal and the other a delayed response from the posterior canal.

Summary

A characteristic nystagmus profile of benign paroxysmal positional nystagmus (BPPN) was determined from analyses of horizontal and vertical electro-oculographic recordings in 8 patients. The vertical component was upbeat in both eyes (fast phase toward the ground in the head-hanging position) while the horizontal component was dissociated with the ipsilateral eye beating away from the down ear and the contralateral eye beating toward the down ear. The amplitude of the vertical component was larger in the contralateral eye while that of the horizontal component was larger in the ipsilateral eye. This dissociated nystagmus profile is consistent with a burst of excitatory activity originating in the posterior canal of the ear that is undermost at the end of the positioning maneuver.

References

1   Dix, M.R. and Hallpike, C.S.: Pathology, symptomatology and diagnosis of certain disorders of the vestibular system. Proc. R. Soc. Med. *45:* 341–354 (1952).
2   Schuknecht, H.: Cupulolithiasis. Archs Otolar. *90:* 765–778 (1969).
3   Sills, A.; Baloh, R.W., and Honrubia, V.: Caloric testing. II. Results in normal subjects. Ann. Otol. Rhinol. Lar. *86:* suppl. 43, pp. 7–23 (1977).
4   Ito, M.: The vestibulo-cerebellar relationships: vestibulo-ocular reflex arc and flocculus; in Naunton, The vestibular system, pp. 129–146 (Academic Press, New York 1975).
5   Cohen, B.; Suzuki, J., and Bender, M.B.: Eye movements from semicircular canal nerve stimulation in the cat. Ann. Otol. Rhinol. Lar. *73:* 153–169 (1964).
6   Fernandez, C.; Alzate, R., and Lindsay, J.R.: Experimental observations on postural nystagmus in the cat. Ann. Otol. Rhinol. Lar. *68:* 816–830 (1959).
7   Allen, G. and Fernandez, C.: Experimental observations in postural nystagmus. I. Extensive lesions in posterior vermis of the cerebellum. Acta oto-lar. *51:* 2–14 (1960).

8 Fernandez, C.; Alzate, R., and Lindsay, J.R.: Interrelations between flocculonodular lobe and vestibular system; in Rasmussen and Windle, Neural mechanisms of the auditory and vestibular systems, pp. 285–296 (Thomas, Springfield 1960).

9 Robinson, D.A.: Oculomotor control signals; in Lennerstrand and Bach-Y-Rita, Mechanisms of ocular motility and their clinical implications (Pergamon Press, Oxford 1975).

10 Baarsma, E.A. and Collewwijn, H.: Eye movements due to linear accelerations in the rabbit. J. Physiol. 245: 227 (1975).

R.W. Baloh, MD, University of California, The Center for the Health Sciences, School of Medicine, Department of Neurology, Los Angeles, CA 90024 (USA)

Adv. Oto-Rhino-Laryng., vol. 25, pp. 167–172 (Karger, Basel 1979)

On the Mechanism of Vestibular Disturbances Caused by Industrial Solvents[1]

L.M. Ödkvist, B. Larsby, R. Tham and G. Aschan

Departments of Otolaryngology and Clinical Pharmacology,
Linköping University, Linköping

Introduction

The vestibular system in man and other mammals is disturbed by ethyl alcohol, which is shown by a positional nystagmus and diminishing of the nystagmus responses to rotatory acceleration. The direction of the positional alcohol nystagmus (PAN) is left beating in a left lateral position and vice versa [*Aschan,* 1958]. Industrial solvents are known to cause fatigue, dizziness and vertigo. Given to rabbits they cause a positional nystagmus with a beat direction the opposite of PAN. As this was first noted for xylene we name it positional xylene nystagmus (PXN) [*Aschan et al.,* 1977]. It has been observed during exposure to xylene, styrene, trichloroethylene and methylchloroform [*Larsby et al.,* 1978 a, b; *Ödkvist et al.,* 1977], all of them causing the same type of nystagmus. In order to investigate the mechanism by which these solvents act on the vestibular system, comparison were made between the action on the vestibular system by three different alcohols, four organic solvents, and some drugs with different action on the central nervous system, i.e. barbiturates, α-chloralose, picrotoxin and bicuculline.

Methods

Rabbits, body weights 2–4 kg, were mounted in a box as described by *Larsby et al.* [1978a]. Electronystagmogram was recorded in upright and lateral positions and during rotatory acceleration.

[1] This research was supported by the Swedish Work Environment Fund, project 75–34 and the Swedish Medical Research Council, grant 17X-0462.

Table I. For three alcohols, four solvents and three drugs known to have an effect on the central nervous system are given the minimal concentration that elicits a recorded vestibular disturbance, the type of positional nystagmus, and the influence by the drug on the nystagmus response to rotatory acceleration

	Minimal concentration, ppm	Nystagmus type	Rotatory response
Methanol	900	PAN	inhibited
Ethanol	500	PAN	inhibited
Propanol	900	PAN	inhibited
Xylene	30	PXN	exaggerated
Styrene	40	PXN	paradoxical
Trichloroethylene	30	PXN	insignificant
Methylchloroform	70	PXN	insignificant
Barbiturates	n.d.	0	inhibited
α-Chloralose	n.d.	PXN	exaggerated
Picrotoxin-bicuculline	n.d.	PXN	insignificant

n.d. = Not determined.

Solutions in 0.9% NaCl of methanol (20%), ethanol (20%), propanol (20–40%), pentobarbital (Nembutal®; 25–50 mg/ml), amobarbital (Isomyl-sodium®, 25–50 mg/ml), α-chloralose (5 mg/ml at 40°C), picrotoxin (0.1 mg/ml) and bicuculline (0.1 mg/ml) were prepared. Styrene and trichloroethylene were dissolved in Intralipid® (10%), as described by *Aschan et al.* [1977]. Most of the drugs were given by intravenous infusion, usually for 1 h. The infusion rates were for methanol 10–24 mg/min/kg, for ethanol 9–20 mg/min/kg, for propanol 9–30 mg/min/kg, for Nembutal® 0.2–0.5 mg/min/kg, for Isomyl-sodium® 0.2–0.5 mg/min/kg, for trichloroethylene 0.2–3.8 mg/min/kg and for styrene 0.2–3.8 mg/min/kg. Picrotoxin and bicuculline were given intravenously during 1–2 min, the total administered amount was 0.6 and 0.08 mg/kg. α-Chloralose was administered intraperitoneally, the total dose being 30–45 mg/kg. For analysis arterial blood and in some experiments cerebrospinal fluid was collected as described by *Larsby et al.* [1978a]. The level of methanol, ethanol, propanol, styrene and trichloroethylene were estimated by gas chromatography.

Results

Methanol, ethanol, propanol all elicited a nystagmus left beating in the left lateral position and vice versa (PAN). Table I summarizes the minimum concentration of the drugs in blood necessary to elicit a positional nystagmus.

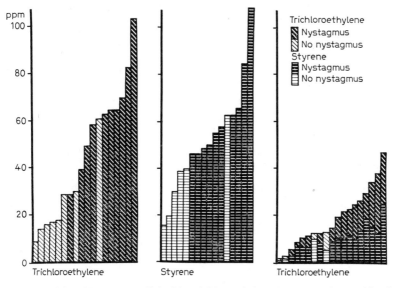

Fig. 1. Positional nystagmus elicited by trichloroethylene, styrene and a combination of them. Each dark bar represents one rabbit experiment resulting in a nystagmus; each light bar an experiment with no nystagmus. The height of the bars indicates the blood concentration of the solvents in parts per million (ppm).

In some experiments ethanol was administered simultaneously with trichloroethylene. At blood levels below 500 ppm (mg/kg of blood) neither did ethanol potentiate nor antagonize the effect of trichloroethylene, i.e. a nystagmus of the PXN-type always appeared at trichloroethylene blood levels above 30 ppm. On the other hand the presence of trichloroethylene at blood levels from 20 to 70 ppm did not interfere with the effect of ethanol, i.e. a nystagmus of the PAN type always appeared at ethanol blood levels above 500–1,000 ppm.

In 11 experiments barbiturates (Nembutal ® or Isomyl-sodium ®) were given by intravenous infusion, usually with a rate causing unconsciousness after about 1 h of infusion. Positional nystagmus never developed, although some nystagmus appeared in an upright position, more of the type gaze nystagmus (table I.)

In 8 experiments α-chloralose was given in amounts which did not affect the consciousness of the rabbits. Six rabbits developed PXN. In 12 experiments bicuculline or picrotoxin were given in nonconvulsive amounts. PXN appeared in 4 out of 5 bicuculline experiments and 5 out of 7 picrotoxin experiments. The effect on the rotatory vestibular response by all the drugs is indicated in table I.

In 18 experiments styrene and trichloroethylene were administered simultaneously. Figure 1 shows that the blood concentrations of trichloroethylene and styrene necessary to elicit a positional nystagmus when administered together are very small compared to the experiments with styrene or trichloroethylene alone. A potentiating action is clearly demonstrated.

The quotient between the cerebrospinal fluid level and the blood level of trichloroethylene or styrene has previously been estimated. Simultaneous administration of both drugs did not change this relationship – the quotients were still 0.05–0.1 for each solvent.

Discussion

PAN is considered to be elicited in the periphery of the vestibular system, i.e. the semicircular canals and be due to the specific weight of the ethyl alcohol [*Money et al.,* 1974]. Other alcohols accordingly give the same type of nystagmus (table I) at about the same blood concentration. Styrene, xylene, trichloroethylene and methylchloroform all elicit a PXN at blood concentrations ten times lower than the one necesarry for alcohol to elicit PAN. This is not due to the specific weight, as indicated by trichloroethylene and methylchloroform having a specific weight above one, xylene and styrene below one. This independence of the specific weight concerning the solvents indicates that PAN and PXN are elicitated by different mechanisms. The experiments with simultaneous administration of ethanol and trichloroethylene support this postulation.

Previous results have suggested that PXN is elicited by a central mechanism [*Aschan et al.,* 1977; *Larsby et al.,* 1978a]. We have therefore investigated the effect of other drugs acting on the central nervous systems. Barbiturates, which represent a group of drugs considered to have a non-selective depressive action on the central nervous system, did not elicit a positional nystagmus. Although α-chloralose is used as an anesthetic, the drug enhances many central reactions, for example the evoked responses in a number of subcortical regions as well as in the cortex [*Borbély,* 1973]. This stimulatory effect is generally regarded as resulting from blockage of inhibitory mechanisms. α-chloralose elicited a PXN, and the same effect had accordingly picrotoxin and biciculline, known to cause a general stimulation of the central nervous system. These results and the previously described effects on the rotatory nystagmus by the organic solvents suggest that the solvents elicit PXN by a selective or nonselective stimulation of the central vestibular pathways, possibly by blocking the inhibition effect from, for example, the reticular formation or the cerebellum. In this connection it is interesting to note that picrotoxin and bicuculline are inhibitors of the γ-aminobutyric acid (GABA). There is strong evidence that this transmitter is involved in the cerebellar inhibition of the vestibular pathways [*Precht et al.,* 1973; *Roffler-Tarlov and Tarlov,* 1975].

The question arises if the similar effect exerted by xylene, styrene, methylchloroform and trichloroethylene is a common mechanism, for example due to their physical properties. If that were the case they could be expected to have a purely additive effect if they were given simultaneously, but our experiments show a 6–8 times potentiation when they were administered together (fig. 1). This potentiation is possibly not pharmacokinetically caused, as simultaneous estimation of their concentration in the cerebrospinal fluid does not unveil any interaction of their penetration into the extracellular space of the central nervous system. The theory of an identical way of action for the solvents is furthermore contradicted by the fact that the solvents have different effects on the rotatory nystagmus responses. (table I). Our conclusion is that these organic solvents affect the central vestibular pathways by different mechanisms.

The potentiating effect in the acute combination experiments suggests that different solvents appearing simultaneously in a working environment could be more poisonous than a higher concentration of a single solvent. This would be of great importance for the occupational medicine. Working with one solvent at a time would be less dangerous than using mixtures, which at present is very common. Further research in these matters appear to be of greatest importance. Theoretical and practical interests are joined.

Summary

The industrial solvents xylene, styrene, trichloroethylene and methylchloroform administered to rabbits caused a positional nystagmus and disturbances in the nystagmus response to rotatory acceleration. The positional nystagmus had a beat direction the opposite to positional alcohol nystagmus, which was in similar experiments elicited by methanol, ethanol and propanol. The three alcohols needed a ten times higher blood concentration to cause a nystagmus than the solvents did.

For comparison, other rabbits were given drugs known to have effects on the central nervous system, depressants and stimulants. The conclusions drawn from the experiments are that the solvents and alcohols have different ways of action. The solvents seem to abolish inhibitions in the central vestibular pathways. A strong potentiating action between solvents is a new finding with importance for occupational medicine.

References

Aschan, G.: Different types of alcohol nystagmus. Acta oto-lar., suppl. 140 (1958).

Aschan, G.; Bunnfors, I.; Hydán, D.; Larsby, B.; Ödkvist, L.M., and Tham, R.: Xylene exposure. Electronystagmographic and gaschromatographic studies in rabbits. Acta oto-lar. *84:* 370–376 (1977).

Borbély, A.: Pharmacological modifications of evoked brain potentials (Huber, Bern 1973).

Larsby, B.; Ödkvist, L.M.; Hydén, D., and Liedgren, S.R.C.: Disturbances of the vestibular system by toxic agents. Acta physiol. Scand., suppl. 440. p. 108 (1976).

Larsby, B.; Tham, R.; Ödkvist, L.M.; Hydén, D.; Bunnfors, I., and Aschan, G.: Exposure of rabbits to styrene. Electronystagmographic findings correlated to the blood and cerebrospinal fluid styrene levels. Scand. J. Work Envir. Hlth *4:* 60–65 (1978a).

Larsby, B.; Tham, R.; Ödkvist, L.M.; Norlander, B.; Aschan, G., and Rubin, A.: Exposure of rabbits to methylchloroform. Vestibular disturbances correlated to blood and cerebrospinal fluid levels. Int. Archs occup. envir. Hlth *41:* 7–15 (1978b).

Money, K.E.; Myles, W.S., and Hoffert, B.M.: The mechanism of positional alcohol nystagmus. Can. J. Otolar. *3:* 302–313 (1974).

Ödkvist, L.M.; Larsby, B., and Liedgren, S.R.C.: Influence of industrial solvents on the vestibular system. XIth Wld Congr. in Otorhinolaryngology, Buenos Aires 1977.

Precht, W.; Baker, R., and Okada, Y.: Evidence for GABA as the synaptic transmitter of the inhibitory vestibuloocular pathway. Expl. Brain. Res. *18:* 415–428 (1973).

Roffler-Tarlov, S. and Tarlov, E.: Studies of suspected neurotransmitters in the vestibuloocular pathways. Brain Res. *95:* 383–394 (1975).

L.M. Ödkvist, MD, Department of Otolaryngology,
Linköping University, Linköping (Sweden)

Adv. Oto-Rhino-Laryng., vol. 25, pp. 173–177 (Karger, Basel 1979)

The Effects of Some Drugs on the Caloric Induced Nystagmus

S. Vesterhauge and E. Peitersen

ENT University Department, Copenhagen Municipal Hospital, Copenhagen

Introduction

Several authors have tested how drugs with effects on vestibular disorders modify experimentally induced nystagmus in normal subjects. Results usually are incomparable because of different methods and evaluations of results. The aim of this work is by means of a standardized method to compare the effects of some different drugs on the caloric-induced nystagmus of normal subjects. The drugs were selected with consideration to their use in the treatment of motion sickness and dizziness of peripheral origin. It has been our aim to cover a spectrum as wide as possible seen from both the clinical and the general pharmacological view.

Material and Methods

30 healthy medical students joined the study. No other medication was allowed during the experimental period. 250 ml of water at 30 °C was used as a stimulus. During the nystagmus recording, using the ENG technique, the subjects performed mental arithmetic. Each student participated in a series of experiments, where different drugs were given at different doses. Each series of tests was opened and closed with caloric control test. Caloric tests were done 10, 20 and 30 min after administration of the drugs. In some drugs (cyclizine, thiethylperazine and metoclopramide) the 10-min stimulus was omitted. Each drug was tested on 5 students. All drugs were given parenterally.

The effects of the drugs were evaluated as the percentual change of the response in relation to the control test responses. The *duration* of the response was measured and the *maximum eye speed (MES) of the slow component* was calculated as the amplitude frequency product of 10 sec of the culmination. We consider this product as a simple and usable expression of the speed of the slow component in cases where the result is expressed as a relation between two single test results [7].

Results

Anticholinergic Drugs. Atropine and *scopolamine* were tested. In contrast to scopolamine, atropine is averse to depress the CNS [4]. The protection index (PI) against motion sickness according to *Holling* [3] of atropine has never been determined to more than 50%. *Wood et al.* [9] calculated the mean PI of scopolamine to 63% referring to 22 authors. *Wood and Graybiel* [8] found that scopolamine was the most protective of all drugs tested against experimentally induced motion sickness. Several handbooks recommend both drugs in the treatment of the acute Meniere attack, but no clinical documentation is accessible. Atropine was given in three doses, 0.5, 1.0 and 2.0 mg. The results appear in figure 1. Both parameters are equally depressed.

Central Nervous System Stimulants. Two drugs were tested, *amphetamine* and *caffeine. Wood and Graybiel* [8] demonstrated that amphetamine was one of the most effective antimotion sickness drugs. Caffeine is commonly used in antimotion sickness preparations to counteract the sedative actions of other drugs, its own efficiency against motion sickness has never been tested. In its central stimulant actions, it resembles amphetamine, though its mechanisms of action differs from that of amphetamine. None of the drugs has been recommended as antivertiginous drugs. The results appear in figure 1. 10 mg of amphetamine gave no significant change, whereas 15 mg significantly prolonged the duration. The results of 150 and 300 mg of caffeine resembles that of amphetamine, though no dose-response relation can be demonstrated.

Antihistamines and Other Antiemetic Drugs. This group of drugs includes some of the classic antimotion sickness and antivertiginous drugs. *Cyclizine* has been chosen as a representative of the piperazines (others are meclizine and cinnarizine). *Thiethylperazine* and *promethazine* are both phenothiazines with very different sedative effects. *Brand and Perry* [1] calculated the mean PI of cyclizine from the literature to 59%, the corresponding value of promethazine being 58%. *Wood et al.* [9] found higher mean values, 71 and 64%, respectively. *Wood and Graybiel* [8] proved that promethazine is the most effective drug in this group, more effective than cyclizine and almost as effective as scopolamine. Thiethylperazine made their subjects more sensitive to motion sickness than placebo. In contrast to this, it is possible to calculate a PI of thiethylperazine of 68% from a

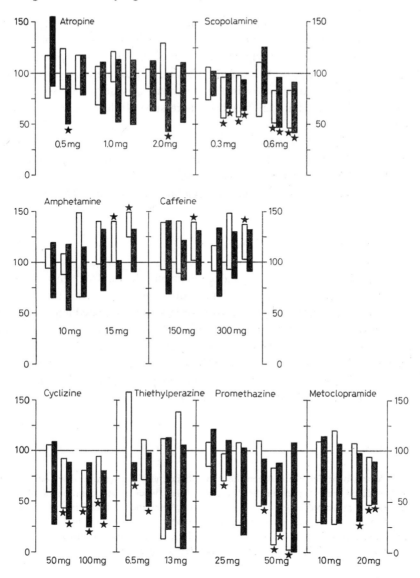

Fig. 1. White columns indicate the mean ± SD of durations, black columns indicate mean ± SD of mes values. Asterisks indicate results significantly different from 100% (p<0.05).

work by *Rubensohn* [6]. All drugs mentioned have been recommended for the treatment of dizziness, only proven in a double-blind study of *Diamant* [2] in the case of thiethylperazine. *Metoclopramide* is a procainamide derivate effective against nausea and vomiting of different origin. Different authors recommend the drug in the treatment of vestibular disorders, but no controlled clinical trial has been accessible. It has no antihistaminic activity.

All drugs in this group were given in the dose usually recommended and twice this dose. The results appear in figure 1. All drugs decreased the response of both parameters. In cyclizine, the subjects seem to be affected in the less variable way. The effect resembles that of scopolamine.

Conclusion

The clinical pharmacological conclusions drawn from this work are rather negative. Well-documented antimotion sickness drugs either suppress or facilitate the caloric response. More or less undocumented antivertiginous drugs like antihistamines suppress the vestibular response, but a drug like apomorphine has been demonstrated [5] to possess a similar ability – and who would ever dream of using this drug in the treatment of vestibular disorders. Thus, the method seems unfit for preclinical evaluation of anti-motion sickness and antivertiginous drugs.

Summary

A striking difference between the two anticholinergic drugs was observed. Atropine only modified the eye speed of the slow phase (mes), whereas scopolamine modified both parameters measured, mes and duration. Amphetamine and caffeine prolonged the duration, leaving the mes unchanged. All antiemetic drugs inhibited both parameters. It is concluded that the effect of a drug on the caloric reaction gives insufficient information in the preclinical evaluation of vestibulo-suppressive drugs.

References

1   Brand, J.J. and Perry, L.M.: Drugs used in motion sickness. Pharmac. Rev. *18:* 895–924 (1966).
2   Diamant, M.: Ett antiemetikum med antivertiginös verkan. Sv. Läkartidn. *61:* 2632–2641 (1964).

3   Holling, H.E.: Prevention of seasickness by drugs. Lancet *i:* 127–129 (1944).
4   Inncs, I.R. and Nickerson, M.: Atropine, scopolamine and related antimuscarinic drugs; in Goodman and Gillman, The pharmacological basic of therapeutics; 5th ed., pp. 514–532 (Macmillan, New York 1975).
5   Peitersen, E.; Fenger, H.J.; Gudmand-Høyer, E., and Vesterhauge, S.: The acoustico-vestibular function during dumping provocation. Acta oto-lar. *73:* 4–9 (1972).
6   Rubensohn, G.: Tietylperazin som profylax och terapi. Sv. Läkartidn. *67:* 619–624 (1970).
7   Vesterhauge, S. and Kildegaard Larsen, P.: Normal values in a routine ENG test. Acta oto-lar. *84:* 91–97 (1977).
8   Wood, C.D. and Graybiel, A.: Evaluation of sixteen antimotion sickness drugs under controlled laboratory condition. Aerospace Med. *39:* 1341–1344 (1968).
9   Wood, C.D.; Kennedy, R.E.; Graybiel, A.; Trumbull, R., and Wherry, R.J.: Clinical effectiveness of antimotion sickness drugs. J. Am. med. Ass. *198:* 133–136 (1966).

S. Vesterhauge, MD, ENT University Department 2071, Rigshospitalet, DK-2100 Copenhagen Ø (Denmark)

Adv. Oto-Rhino-Laryng., vol. 25, pp. 178–183 (Karger, Basel 1979)

Effect of Ethacrynic Acid upon the Peripheral Vestibular Nystagmus

J. Kusakari, Y. Sato, T. Kobayashi, S. Saijo and K. Kawamoto

Department of Otolaryngology, Tohoku University School of Medicine, Sendai

Introduction

Kusakari and Thalmann [1] reported that the endolymphatic potential in the guinea pig ampulla (AEP) was reduced by anoxia or i.v. administration of ethacrynic acid (ETA). These results indicate that the AEP has a positive component which is probably produced by an active transport mechanism. The purpose of the present experiment is to determine what happens on the nystagmus of peripheral vestibular origin when the AEP is reduced by ETA.

Materials and Methods

61 albino guinea pigs weighing 250–350 g were used. ETA solution (Na-ethacrynate, MSD) was given i.v. over a period of 3 min through the indwelling catheter in the neck vein. Nystagmus was recorded by ENG (time constant: 3.0 and 0.03) and the observation was made for 3 h after the administration of ETA. 3 ml of physiological saline solution was injected in control animals.

Unilateral labyrinthectomy. After mechanical destruction of the labyrinth under local anesthesia, a few drops of 90% alcohol was put into the inner ear. ETA was given 30 min after the appearance of nystagmus toward the opposite ear.

Pendular Rotation. An amplitude was 120° and a period 8 sec. Number of nystagmus beats in each cycle was counted.

Galvanic Stimulation. The right ear was stimulated by a cathodic galvanic current of about 2 mA with the unipolar uniaural method. Stimulation was done for 20 sec, and the eye movement was recorded using a photoelectronystagmography. The effect of 100 mg/kg ETA was examined in 3 animals with 3 controls.

Bechterew's Compensatory Nystagmus. About 2 weeks after the first unilateral labyrinthectomy, the opposite ear was destroyed and the nystagmus toward the initially destroyed ear was elicited. 100 mg/kg ETA was given in 3 animals with 4 controls.

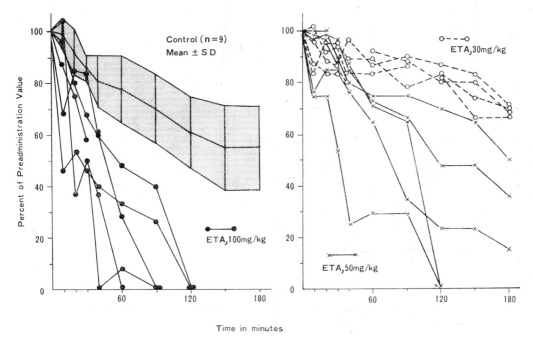

Fig. 1. Effect of ETA upon the nystagmus after unilateral labyrinthectomy (number of nystagmus beats).

Optokinetic Nystagmus. A optokinetic drum (Ohm type) was used at a drum speed of 30°/sec. 3 animals were given 100 mg/kg ETA with 3 controls.

EEG. EEG was recorded in the parietal and the occipital area, and the effect of 100 mg/kg ETA was examined in 3 animals.

Results

Paralytic Nystagmus After Unilateral Labyrinthectomy. 30, 50 and 100 mg/kg ETA were given in 2, 5 and 5 animals, respectively, and the physiological saline solution was given in 9 control animals. The total number of nystagmus beats for 30 sec was counted at various times after the administration, and the number was compared with the preadministration value. As is shown in figure 1, the reduction of the nystagmus beats was significantly greater in 100 mg/kg ETA given animals than the control. In 50 mg/kg group, 2 animals showed no difference from the control but the other 3 showed larger reduction than the control. No statistical difference

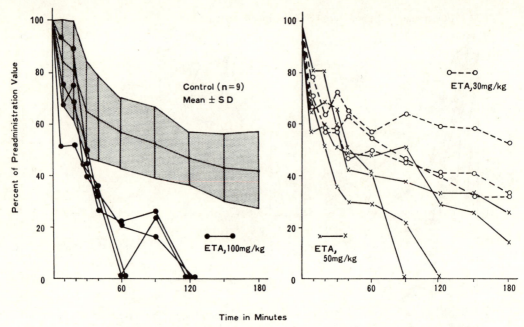

Time in Minutes

Fig. 2. Effect of ETA upon the nystagmus after unilateral labyrinthectomy (slow phase velocity).

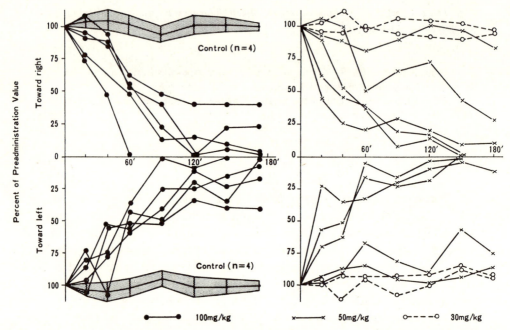

Fig. 3. Effect of ETA upon the nystagmus provoked by a pendular rotation.

was found between 30 mg/kg ETA given animals and the control. The effects of ETA upon the slow phase velocity of the nystagmus was almost identical to those upon the number of the nystagmus beats (fig. 2).

Pendular Rotation Nystagmus. No habituation or adaptation of nystagmus was observed in 4 control animals. 100 mg/kg ETA given animals exhibited a remarkable reduction in number of the nystagmus beats. 50 mg/kg ETA produced a strong inhibition in 3 animals, whereas milder or no inhibition occurred in 2. 30 mg/kg ETA had no effect upon pendular rotation nystagmus (fig. 3).

Others. There was no significant effect of 100 mg/kg ETA upon galvanic nystagmus, Bechterew's compensatory nystagmus, optokinetic nystagmus and EEG.

Discussion

The present experiment shows that ETA inhibits the nystagmus of peripheral vestibular origin. Experiments along this line using the cat were reported by *Levinson et al.* [2] and *Mathog* [3]. They also reported that ETA inhibited the nystagmus response to caloric irrigation, although the mode of action and dose-response relation were different from ours probably due to the different sensitivity to ETA between the cat and the guinea pig. It is evident that when 100 mg/kg ETA was given in guinea pigs, AEP becomes negative in about 30 min and exhibits the maximal depression in about 1.5 h [1]. This progressive change of the potential is quite similar to that of peripheral vestibular nystagmus [1]. These results strongly suggest that the inhibition of the peripheral vestibular nystagmus by ETA is mainly due to the reduction of the AEP.

One discrepancy exists between the AEP experiment and the present one. Namely, in the AEP experiment the dosage of ETA which reduced the AEP is 60 mg/kg or greater, and 50 mg/kg ETA did not reduce the AEP. However, in some animals given 50 mg/kg ETA the nystagmus of the peripheral vestibular origin was inhibited in the present experiment. The question then arises whether this discrepancy is only due to the different experimental conditions between two experiments or there is another site in the vestibular system which is concurrently affected and more sensitive to ETA than the production site of AEP. There are several possible explanations for this phenomenon. One possible explanation is the involvement of the otolith organ. *Sellick et al.* [4], however, reported that 42–66 mg/kg ETA did not have any effect upon the utricular endolymphatic potential. The saccule is another possible candidate but presently there are no available reports. Another possibility is sensory hair cell damage. Although *Quick and Duvall* [5] observed no alternations of vestibular structure in guinea pigs given up to 86 mg/kg, it is still difficult to determine whether the sensory hair cells are affected by ETA or not. In the present experiment, no effect of ETA was observed upon galvanic nystagmus, Bechterew's compensatory nystagmus, OKN or EEG. Although the site of galvanic stimulation is one of the most controversial questions in vestibular physiology, the most provable site seems to be the Scarpa's ganglion or the vestibular nerve [6]. Bechterew's compensatory nystagmus is due to the activity of the vestibular nucleus on the side of the labyrinth first destroyed. Abnormality of OKN is known to occur in the disorders of the occulomotor or central vestibular system. In the present experiment, we could not obtain any result suggesting that ETA has any effect on the vestibular nerve, Scarpa's ganglion or CNS. One more possible explanation is the effect of ETA upon the corneo-retinal potential. But this is not the case because 100 mg/kg ETA did not have any effect upon the slow phase velocity of optokinetic nystagmus. The last but not the least possible is the difference in the experimental conditions. In the AEP experiment, the animal was anesthetized by pentobarbital and artificially respired after administration of gallamine triethiodide, whereas the animal was mentally alert in the present experiment. This difference in the experimental condition may have caused the previously mentioned discrepancy.

Recent studies by many investigators [7, 8] indicate that the production of the endolymph and the maintenance of its characteristic ionic composition intimately relates to the production of the endolymphatic potential. Although several other auxiliary causes may exist, it is reasonable to assume from the present experiment that the inhibition of the peripheral vestibular nystagmus is mainly due to the reduction of the AEP. It is our conclusion that the presence of a normal AEP is a prerequisite to the maintenance of a normal vestibular function.

Summary

The effect of ethacrynic acid (ETA) upon pendular rotation nystagmus and paralytic nystagmus was examined using 61 guinea pigs. 100 mg/kg ETA reduced these nystagmus but 30 mg/kg ETA had on effect. Galvanic nystagmus, Bechterew's compensatory nystagmus, OKN and EEG were not affected by 100 mg/kg ETA. These results are highly suggestive that the inhibition of the peripheral vestibular nystagmus by ETA is mainly due to the reduction of the ampullar endolymphatic potential.

References

1   Kusakari, J. and Thalmann, R.: Effects of anoxia and ethacrynic acid upon ampullar endolymphatic potential and upon high energy phosphates in ampullar wall. Laryngoscope 86: 132–147 (1976).
2   Levinson, R.M.; Capps, M.J., and Mathog, R.H.: Ethacrynic acid. furosemide and vestibular caloric responses. Ann. Otol. Rhinol. Lar. 83: 223–229 (1974).
3   Mathog, R.H.: Vestibulotoxicity of ethacrynic acid. Laryngoscope 87: 1791–1808 (1977).
4   Sellick, P.M.; Johnstone, J.R., and Johnstone, B.M.: The electrophysiology of the utricle. Pflügers Arch. ges. Physiol. 336: 21–27 (1972).
5   Quick, C.A. and Duvall, A.J.: Early changes in the cochlear duct from ethacrynic acid: an electronmicroscopic evaluation. Laryngoscope 80: 954–965 (1970).
6   Pfaltz, C.R.: The diagnostic importance of the galvanic test in otoneurology. ORL 31: 193–203 (1969).
7   Kuijpers, W.: Cation transport and cochlear function, thesis University of Nijmegen (1969).
8   Bosher, S.R.; Smith, C., and Warren, R.L.: The effects of ethacrynic acid upon the cochlear endolymph and the stria vascularis. Acta oto-lar. 75: 184–191 (1973).

J. Kusakari, MD, Department of Otolaryngology,
Tohoku University School of Medicine, Sendai (Japan)

Adv. Oto-Rhino-Laryng., vol. 25, pp.184–191 (Karger, Basel 1979)

Vestibular Neuronal Function during Ischemia

Response of Vestibular Neurons to Vertebral and
Carotid Artery Occlusion in Rabbits

T. Matsunaga, M. Sano, K. Yamamoto and T. Kubo

Department of Otolaryngology, Osaka University Medical School, Osaka

Introduction

In contrast to the susceptibility of cochlear functions to ischemia or
anoxia, which has been studied extensively by many investigators such as
Maruyama [1956], *Sugano* [1960], *Lawrence et al.* [1975] and *Makishima
et al.* [1976], the susceptibility of vestibular functions has defied exploration
because it is lacking in suitable indicators, as likened by cochlear potentials
which faithfully reflect cochlear functions.

The authors reported in previous papers that vertiginous patients suffer
from disturbed blood flow in vertebral and common carotid arteries with
the use of Doppler's ultrasonic flowmeter [*Matsunaga et al.,* 1974, 1975],
and have analyzed the relation between ischemia produced by occlusion of
these arteries and vestibular excitability in rabbits.

This paper is concerned with a study of neuronal activities in the
vestibular nuclei altered by complete or partial occlusion of vertebral and
common carotid arteries.

Material and Methods

The vertebral and common carotid arteries of 20 healthy adult rabbits were exposed
by a midline cervical incision, with the animals in supine position and under nembutal
anesthesia. A silk thread was looped around these arteries for occlusion. The animals
were tracheotomized for artificial respiration, and immobilized by gallamine in a prone
position with the head fixed on a stereotaxic frame. The animals were then placed on the
center of a turntable for sinusoidal rotation in the horizontal plane.

The vestibular nucleus neurons were provided with a glass microelectrode, which
was carefully inserted with the aid of a stereotaxic instrument and a brain atlas, to record

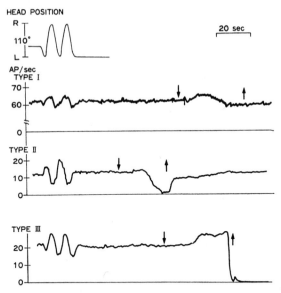

Fig. 1. Three different patterns of alteration of vestibular neuronal activity during occlusion of vestibular arteries are shown.

their unitary activity. The frequency of neuronal discharge was measured with a pulse counter and recorded with a pen recorder in the manner presented in our previous papers [*Matsunaga et al.,* 1975; *Kubo et al.,* 1977]. Complete occlusion and partial occlusion of the blood flow were achieved by pulling the thread and loading weights of 15, 30 and 45 g on the arteries during about 60–180 sec.

In some animals a monopolar silver stimulation electrode was inserted into an inner ear through the round window according to Fredrickson's method [*Fredrickson et al.,* 1966] to record field potentials evoked in the vestibular nuclei by the occlusion of vertebral and/or common carotid arteries. A rectangular pulse was delivered with the following parameters:

1 Hz; 0.05–0.1 msec; 5–10 V

The field potentials displayed on an ordinary oscilloscope were continuously photographed on X-films. Successful insertion of the recording electrode in a vestibular nuclei was histologically verified.

Results

Neuronal Activity during Occlusion

A total of 102 vestibular neurons responsive to sinusoidal rotation were examined for changes in activity resulting from occlusion, either ipsilateral,

Table I. Alteration of neuronal activity during occlusion[1]

Type	Vertebral artery			Common carotid artery		
	ipsilateral	contralateral	bilateral	ipsilateral	contralateral	bilateral
I	$25/60$ (42)	$11/42$ (26)	$8/21$ (38)	$2/6$ (25)	$2/8$ (25)	$5/23$ (22)
II	$6/60$ (10)	$3/42$ (7)	$4/21$ (19)	$1/8$ (13)	$1/8$ (13)	$7/23$ (30)
III	$18/60$ (30)	$9/42$ (21)	$6/21$ (29)	$2/8$ (25)	$2/8$ (25)	$7/23$ (30)
Total	$49/60$ (82)	$23/42$ (55)	$18/21$ (86)	$5/8$ (63)	$5/8$ (63)	$19/23$ (82)
IV	$11/60$ (18)	$19/42$ (45)	$3/21$ (14)	$3/8$ (37)	$3/8$ (37)	$4/23$ (18)

[1] The incidence of patterns of altered vestibular neuronal activity during ipsilateral, contralateral and bilateral occlusion of vestibular and common carotid arteries are shown for types I, II and III, see text. Type IV refers to the unaltered activity. Percentages are indicated in parentheses.

contralateral or both, of vertebral or common carotid arteries. The patterns of change in activity of the vestibular neurons before, during and after occlusion were classified into types 1 to 3 according to the frequency of neuronal discharges (fig. 1). Type 1 consisted of a transient increase and gradual return to the initial activity during occlusion. Type 2 consisted of an abrupt or slow decrease and gradual return to the initial level after release of occlusion. Type 3 was made up of a transient increase, abrupt decrease and disappearance of activity during occlusion.

The interval between the beginning of occlusion and the onset of altered activity ranged from about 2 to 60 sec.

Abrupt decreases to nullify the frequency of action potentials were neglected, because such a pattern is ascribable to slightest relative movement of the brain to the recording microelectrode due to pull of threads, which may take place despite operators' utmost effort to prevent it.

The total number of occlusions was 123 for vertebral arteries (ipsilateral, 60; contralateral, 42; bilateral, 21), and 39 for common carotid

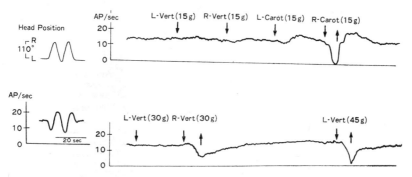

Fig. 2. The alteration of neuronal activity during partial occlusion of the four arteries is shown.

arteries (ipsilateral, 8; contralateral, 8; bilateral, 23) (table I). For occlusion of vertebral arteries, alteration of neuronal activity was detected in 49 (82%) of the 60 occlusions of the ipsilateral artery, in 23 (55%) of the 42 occlusions of the contralateral artery, and in 18 (86%) of the 21 occlusions of bilateral arteries. Therefore, changes in vestibular neuronal activity due to occlusion of the ipsilateral artery differed significantly from those due to occlusion of the contralateral artery.

As for the three different patterns of changes in vestibular neuronal activity, type 1 was the most frequent, and type 3 and type 2, in decreasing order, followed type 1. Meanwhile, the frequency of changes in neuronal activity resulting from occlusion of common carotid arteries nearly equaled that from occlusion of vertebral arteries, though occlusion of common carotid arteries caused little difference between ipsilateral and contralateral arteries in changes of the activity.

Neuronal Activity during Partial Occlusion

The finding that occlusion of a common carotid artery or arteries affects the activity of the vestibular nucleus neurons prompted us to occlude partially the four arteries, i.e. bilateral vertebral and common carotid arteries, in arbitrary order (fig. 2).

A 15 g load on both vertebral arteries and a common carotid artery did not alter neuronal activity, but the same load on the other common carotid artery produced a type 2 pattern change. A 30 g load on a single vertebral artery did not alter the activity, but the same load on the other vertebral artery produced a type 2 pattern. A 45 g load on the ipsilateral vertebral artery also produced a type 2 pattern.

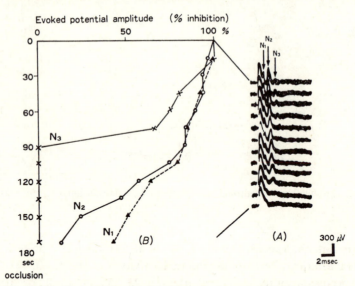

Fig. 3. A Vestibular field potentials. Note the decreased amplitudes during occlusion.
B Percent inhibition of amplitude in negative waves of N_1, N_2 and N_3.

Vestibular Field Potential during Occlusion

Figure 3A shows field potentials produced in the vestibular nuclei by electrical stimulation of an inner ear. N_1 negative waves, which are regarded as presynaptic potentials in the vestibular nuclei, had latency of about 0.75 msec. N_2 waves, which are regarded as monosynaptic potentials, had latency of about 1.5 msec and, N_3 waves as polysynaptic potentials, about 2.3 msec.

In general, amplitudes of the field potentials were unaltered when any of the four arteries remained unoccluded, and it was only after occlusion of all the four arteries that the amplitudes were reduced. In this occasion, reduction of N_1 waves was preceded by that of N_2 and N_3 waves (fig. 3B), and the latency for these waves were found to have been prolonged during occlusion.

Discussion

The authors' observation of the 3 patterns in vestibular neuronal activity during ischemia is connected with the observation of various patterns in cortical neuronal activity by *Heiss et al.* [1976], who reported that alteration of cortical neuronal activity occurs between 10 and 120 sec after beginning occlusion of the middle cerebral artery. In the present experiment, alteration of vestibular neuronal activity occurred about 2–60 sec after beginning occlusion of one vertebral artery, about 2–30 sec after beginning occlusion of bilateral arteries, and still as early as 10 sec or less after occluding the four arteries. Accordingly, the interval between the beginning of occlusion and the onset of altered activity is to depend on the grade of ischemia.

Increases in frequency of neuronal discharge during ischemia, which were observed in type 1 pattern and in the early stage of type 3 pattern, have also been reported by *Przybylski* [1971], *Heiss et al.* [1976] and *Nosaka* [1976], and have been ascribed to frequency increment, which is due to an increase of afferentation from reticular formation, chemoreceptor and a decrease of the inhibitory influence from adjacent cortical neurons, or hyperirritability induced by hypoxia and hypoglycemia.

A separate experiment of ours, in which the blood flow in the vestibular nuclei during occlusion was measured by the thermoclearance method, showed that the changes in the blood flow are divided also into three patterns, and that these patterns do not necessarily correlate with the patterns of change in vestibular neuronal activity.

The authors are convinced that this seeming disparity necessitates further experiments in animals whose general conditions of the animals are carefully assessed.

Occlusion of vertebral arteries caused significant difference between the ipsilateral and contralateral vessels in the resultant change of vestibular neuronal activity, and showed that hemodynamic changes due to occlusion of the ipsilateral artery influence the activity of vestibular neurons more prominently than the changes caused by occlusion of the contralateral artery.

In contrast, occlusion of common carotid arteries caused no significant difference between the right and left vessels in the resultant change of the activity and, to the authors' surprise, differed little, either, from occlusion of vertebral arteries in the incidence of the changes. It is obvious, therefore, that the blood flow to the vestibular nuclei passes the vertebral arteries as well as from the carotid arteries.

Partial occlusion of the four arteries injecting to the brain let the author to confirm the role of Willis' circle in the maintenance of blood flow to the vestibular nuclei. This finding made it clear that, when the blood flow to the vestibular nuclei decreases to a certain critical level [*Nakai et al., 1977*], a slightest occlusion of any of the four arteries can impair the vestibular neuronal activity.

The vulnerability of the central auditory pathway to anoxia was found to be higher than that of the end organ by *Makishima et al.* [1976]. The field potentials in the vestibular nuclei recorded by us were similar to those reported by *Matsuoka* [1972]. The promptness of the reduction in amplitude of the three waves in evoked field potentials during occlusion was in the decreasing order of N_3, N_2 and N_1. This finding supports higher vulnerability of the central vestibular pathway to ischemia.

Summary

The relation between ischemia experimentally produced by occlusion of arteries injecting to the brain and the changes in vestibular excitability was examined in 102 rabbit vestibular neurons responding to sinusoidal rotation. During occlusion of ipsilateral and/or contralateral vertebral and common carotid arteries, the neuronal activity took on three different patterns with respect to the frequency of neuronal discharge.

The incidence of alteration of neuronal activities reflected vestibular excitability dependent on hemodynamic changes due to occlusion of the ipsilateral vertebral artery rather than due to occlusion of the contralateral artery.

Occlusion of common carotid arteries caused no significant difference between the right and left vessels in the resultant change of the neuronal activity, and differed little, either, from occlusion of vertebral arteries in the incidence of the changes.

A supplementary experiment, in which the four arteries were only partially occluded, clearly showed that the resultant changes in neuronal activity reflect the role of Willis' circle in the maintenance of blood flow to vestibular nuclei.

References

Fredrickson, J.M.; Schwarz, D., and Kornhuber, H.H.: Convergence and interaction of vestibular and deep somatic afferents upon neurons in the vestibular nuclei of cat. Acta oto-lar. *61:* 168–188 (1966).

Heiss, W.O.; Hayakawa, T., and Waltz, A.G.: Cortical neuronal function during ischemia, effect of occlusion of one middle cerebral artery on single-unit activity in cats. Archs Neurol. *33:* 813–820 (1976).

Kubo, T.; Matsunaga, T., and Matano, S.: Convergence of ampullar and macular inputs on vestibular nuclei unit of the rat. Acta oto-lar. *84:* 166–177 (1977).

Lawrence, M.; Nuttall, A.L., and Burgio, P.A.: Cochlear potentials and oxygen associated with hypoxia. Ann. Otol. Rhinol. Lar. *84:* 499–512 (1975).

Makishima, K; Katz, R.B., and Snow, J.B.: Hearing loss of a central type secondary to anoxic anoxia. Ann. Otol. Rhinol. Lar. *85:* 826–832 (1976).

Maruyama, N.: Experimental observations on the labyrinthine blood flow and the hearing. Jap. J. Otol. *59:* 717–732 (1956).

Matsunaga, T.; Kawamoto, H.; Okumura, S., and Naito, T.: Ultrasonic blood rheo-
graphy in vertebral artery of vertigo patients (Doppler method) – with the glass
model experiments. Med. J. Osaka Univ. *25:* 43–56 (1974).

Matsunaga, T.; Sano, M., and Kubo, T.: A clinical investigation of vertigo and vertebral blood flow using the ultrasonic Doppler method; in Morimoto, Proc. V. Extraord. Meet. of the Bárány Society, 1975, pp. 228–233.

Matsunaga, T. and Kubo, T.: Influence of the hypothalamic stimulation on vestibular
nuclei units in the rat. Acta oto-lar. *80:* 206–213 (1975).

Matsuoka, I.: Effects of diphenidol on the central nervous system in cats. Pract. Otol.,
Kyoto *65:* 179–187 (1972).

Nakai, K.; Welch, M.A., and Meyer, J.S.: Critical cerebral blood flow for production of
hemiparesis after unilateral carotid occlusion in the gerbil. J. Neurol. Neurosurg.
Psychiat. *40:* 595–599 (1977).

Nosaka, S.: Responses of rat brain stem neurons to carotid occlusion. Am. J. Physiol.
231: 20–27 (1976).

Przybylski, A.: Activity pattern of visceral cortex neurons during asphyxia. Expl. Neurol.
32: 12–21 (1971).

Sugano, T.: Experimental studies of the effect of the blood flow changes on the cochlear microphonics and the action potentials. Jap. J. Otol. *63:* 2015–2040 (1960).

Toru Matsunaga, MD, Department of Otolaryngology,
Osaka University Medical School, 553 Fukushimaku, Osaka (Japan)

Adv. Oto-Rhino-Laryng., vol. 25, pp. 192–196 (Karger, Basel 1979)

Low-Frequency Harmonic Acceleration in the Evaluation of Surgical Treatment of Meniere's Disease[1,2]

James W. Wolfe, Edward J. Engelken and James E. Olson

USAF School of Aerospace Medicine, Brooks AFB, Tex., and Wilford Hall USAF Medical Center, Lackland AFB, Tex.

Introduction

One of the major pathologic entities that the otolaryngologist is often confronted with is Meniere's disease. Although the histopathology and symptoms of this condition have been well known for many years, the choice of treatment in any particular patient is not definite. In those cases where surgery has been performed, clinical symptomatology has been the major criterion for evaluating the efficacy of the procedure and no attempts have been made to determine changes which may occur within structures subversing the vestibulo-oculomotor reflex. Recent studies [5, 6] have indicated that low-frequency harmonic acceleration is a reliable test of vestibulo-oculomotor function. Assuming that endolymphatic surgical procedures cause changes in the fluid dynamics of the labyrinth, it should be possible to show changes in responses to harmonic acceleration following surgical treatment for Meniere's disease. The present study was designed to evaluate pre- and postoperative vestibular responses in patients with typical findings [1] of Meniere's disease. It should be emphasized that the decision to select any patient for surgery was not predicated on the responses to harmonic acceleration.

[1] The research reported in this paper was conducted by personnel of the Clinical Sciences and Biometrics Divisions, USAF School of Aerospace Medicine, Aerospace Medical Division, AFSC, Brooks AFB, Tex. and the Otolaryngology and Neurosurgery Services, Wilford Hall USAF Medical Center, Aerospace Medical Division, AFSC, Lackland AFB, Tex.

[2] The voluntary informed consent of subjects used in this research was obtained in accordance with AFR 80-33.

Materials and Methods

23 patients with the diagnosis of Meniere's disease were tested with harmonic acceleration at 0.01, 0.02, 0.04, 0.08, and 0.16 Hz, with a peak velocity of 50°/sec. The stimuli were generated by a Contraves-Goerz DP-300 torque motor system. Subjects were seated in a light-tight, sound-proofed capsule with the head flexed 30° for maximal stimulation of the horizontal canals. All tests were conducted in the dark with eyes open. Eye movements were recorded by conventional electo-oculographic (EOG) techniques. Nystagmus in response to acceleration was analyzed on-line by analog and digital computer techniques [3]. Measures of the phase relationship of the nystagmic output to the input stimulus and labyrinthine preponderance (left-right-asymmetry) were determined for each stimulus frequency. In addition, all patients were given standard bithermal caloric stimulation. 7 of these patients were selected to receive endolymphatic mastoid shunts [4] for intractable vertigo and/or highly fluctuant hearing loss or a combination of the two. 1 patient eventually had bilateral surgery. These patients were restested 5–9 days postoperatively with harmonic acceleration at the same parameters used preoperatively.

Results

When compared to normal subjects from a previous study [5], the patients with Meniere's disease showed differences in their phase lags at all frequencies except 0.04 Hz. Their absolute labyrinthine preponderance (left-right-asymmetry) showed differences only at the two lowest frequencies. Following endolymphatic mastoid shunts their pooled data (fig. 1 A) showed a decrease in phase lag, at all frequencies, of 2–5° while their labyrinthine preponderance showed a regression toward the normal means.

Figure 1 B shows data from a patient with bilateral Meniere's disease of unknown etiology. A bithermal caloric test showed minimal unilateral weakness (6% right) and a directional preponderance of 20% to the right. However, his caloric responses were highly variable and showed a high slow phase velocity (48°/sec) with cold water in the left ear. His responses to harmonic acceleration showed a significant decrement in phase lag at 0.01 and 0.02 Hz. In addition, he had marked labyrinthine preponderance toward the involved side at all frequencies, suggesting an irritable condition or vestibular recruitment. This patient was retested 9 days following a left endolymphatic shunt; as shown in figure 1 B, he reflected even further decrements in phase lag except at the higher frequencies. His labyrinthine preponderance showed an average overall reduction of 63%. Following his left endolymphatic-mastoid shunt the patient had classical Meniere's disease attacks with fullness, roaring tinnitus and hearing fluctuation in the right ear.

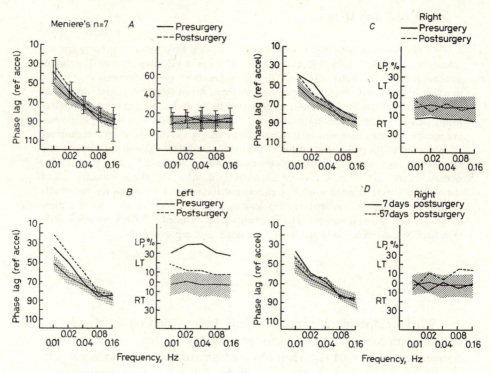

Fig. 1. A Grouped data from 7 patients showing phase shifts and labyrinthine preponderance before and after endolymphatic mastoid shunts. B Data from a patient before
and after a left endolymphatic shunt. C Data from same patient as in figure 1A before
and after a right endolymphatic shunt. D Data from same patient 7 and 57 days postshunt.

2 months after the left shunt his responses to harmonic acceleration showed
a decrease from his previous phase decrements, and he had a labyrinthine
preponderance of 15 % to the right at all frequencies (fig. 1 C). When retested
following a right endolymphatic shunt, he had an improvement in his phase
relationships except at the lowest frequency. There was a marked improvement in his labyrinthine preponderance at all frequencies (to well within
normal limits). This patient had one mild attack which he believed was
related to his left ear 1 month after his surgery. We were able to test him
57 days postoperatively (second procedure) and he showed a slight improvement in his phase shifts with an increase in labyrinthine preponderance
to the left at the higher frequencies (fig. 1 D). 6 months have elapsed since
the second procedure and he is doing quite well clinically.

Discussion

Due to limitations on the length of this paper, it is not possible to present all the relevant findings from this study. One of the more complex cases has been used to demonstrate that endolymphatic hydrops and shunt procedures lead to changes in the fluid dynamics of the semicircular canals. The fact that patients diagnosed as having Meniere's disease show significant low-frequency decrements in their phase relationships is consistent with the mathematic descriptions of canal dynamics [2]. If the diameter of a membranous canal were to increase by 41 % (approximately 0.06 mm), there would be a one octave shift in the lower corner frequency of the response which would be reflected as less phase lag at the lower frequencies.

The fact that the phase can show an even greater transitory decrement following an endolymphatic shunt procedure implies that the pressure is even more affected by manipulation of the sac. It is possible that these changes may be related to electrolytic imbalances within the endolymphatic system which affect hair cell depolarization.

It is evident from the present study that low frequency harmonic acceleration is a sensitive test of canal function and can be used to evaluate the outcome of surgical procedures on the inner ear. Obviously, further studies are needed to clarify the pathophysiology of endolymphatic hydrops and the basis for changes which occur in vestibular responses following shunt procedures.

Summary

23 patients with classical findings of Meniere's disease and so diagnosed by a neurotologist were tested with harmonic acceleration. 7 of these patients were selected to receive endolymphatic-mastoid shunts for intractable vertigo and/or highly progressive fluctuant hearing loss. All 7 patients showed an increase in the impairment in their phase relationships at the lowest frequency (0.01 Hz) following surgery which was considered to be secondary to the procedure. Later this phase lag returned to a level approaching normal. They also showed a definite decrease in the asymmetry (labyrinthine preponderance) of their nystagmic responses to acceleration.

Acknowledgements

The authors wish to acknowledge the editorial assistance and cooperation of *H.H. Hanna,* MD, Chief, Otolaryngology Branch, Brooks AFB, Tex., and the statistical assistance of *Robert J. Fuchs*, Biometrics Division. The authors thank *John W. Docken, Daniel E. Dreher, Norwood E. Gray*, Jr., *La Verne A. Spriggs*, and *D.C. Yount* for their technical assistance.

References

1   Alford, B.R.: Report of subcommittee on equilibrium and its measurement. Trans Am. Acad. Ophthal. Oto-lar. *76:* 1462–1464 (1972).
2   Egmond, A.A.J. van; Groen, J.J., and Jongkees, L.B.W.: The mechanics of the semi-circular canal. J. Physiol. *110:* 1–17 (1949).
3   Engelken, E.J. and Wolfe, J.W.: Analog processing of vestibular nystagmus for on-line cross-correlation data analysis. Aviat. Space environ. Med. *48:* 210–214 (1977).
4   Paparella, M.M. and Hanson, D.G.: Endolymphatic sac drainage for intractable vertigo (method and experiences). Laryngoscope *86:* 697–703 (1976).
5   Wolfe, J.W.; Engelken, E.J., and Kos, C.M.: Low-frequency harmonic acceleration as a test of labyrinthine function: Basic methods and illustrative cases. Trans. Am. Acad. Ophthal. Oto-lar. *86:* 130–142 (1978).
6   Wolfe, J.W.; Engelken, E.J.; Olson, J.E., and Kos, C.M.: Vestibular responses to bithermal caloric and harmonic acceleration. Ann. Otol. Rhinol. Lar. (in press, 1978).

J.W. Wolfe, PhD, School of Aerospace Medicine (NGEV), Brooks AFB, TX 78235 (USA)

Adv. Oto-Rhino-Laryng., vol. 25, pp. 197–201 (Karger, Basel 1979)

Head-Eye Coordination in
Normals and in Patients with Vestibular Disorders

G.R. Barnes

RAF Institute of Aviation Medicine, Farnborough, Hants.

Introduction

In normal human subjects the vestibular system plays an important part in the coordination of head and eye movements during visual search, the compensatory component of the vestibulo-ocular reflex response serving to space-stabilise the eye [4]. Patients with loss of vestibular function might be expected to experience impairment of head-eye coordination, were it not for the adaptation which is known to take place. The nature of this adaptive process has been investigated in a series of experiments in which the oculo-motor responses of normal subjects and of patients with vestibular disorders have been compared.

Slow Phase Eye Movements

Experiment I

Oculomotor responses, in the absence of vision, were compared in a group of 8 normal individuals in 3 experimental conditions: (a) voluntary oscillation of the head, (b) whole body oscillation on a turntable, and (c) stimulation of neck afferents by oscillating the body while fixing the head in space. In each of the experimental conditions the subject sat with the head upright and experienced a sinusoidal angular displacement about the vertical axis with a peak velocity of $\pm 60°$/sec at frequencies between 0.2 and 1.3 Hz.

The response of the eyes during voluntary head movement and whole-body passive movement was very similar, so that at higher frequencies (above 0.8 Hz) there was little difference in the gain and phase of the vestibular reflex. At lower frequencies (0.2–0.8 Hz) the voluntary movement, on average, produced a slightly higher gain, but there was no significant difference because of the considerable intersubject variance. There was little asymmetry in the slow phase velocity of the sinusoidally modulated nystagmus, the mean difference between peak velocity to the left and to the right (fig. 1), here defined as the directional preponderance (DP), having a mean value of $0.08°/sec$ (SD $1.88°/sec$).

The response of the cervico-ocular reflex was not stereotyped, the eye movements of each subject falling into one of three categories [3]: (a) low amplitude slow phase movements which were approximately compensatory for the relative movement between head and body, sometimes interspersed with irregular saccadic activity, (b) eye movements with negligible slow phase activity but regular saccadic activity producing an approximately compensatory eye displacement, and (c) large amplitude pendular eye movements which were difficult to classify as fast or slow phases. Differences in gain between the vestibulo-ocular response to active and passive stimuli for each subject could not be attributed directly to the amplitude of the cervico-ocular response.

Experiment II

All the tests outlined above were also carried out on a group of 11 patients with unilateral loss of vestibular function arising as a result of surgical procedures for the treatment of vestibular disorders. 7 of the patients, for whom there were no pre-operative data, had been labyrinthectomised between 6 months and 20 years prior to the tests. The remaining 4 patients were tested both pre- and post-operatively.

The results of the tests revealed no significant difference from the normal population in the gain and phase of either the vestibulo-ocular or cervico-ocular reflex, although 4 patients examined both pre- and post-operatively showed a significant decrease (mean 22 %) in gain of the vestibular reflex after labyrinthectomy. The most important feature, however, was a marked asymmetry of the nystagmic response during both voluntary and passive head movement. There was a directional preponderance of the sinusoidally modulated slow phase velocity towards the side of the lesion, which was significantly greater ($p < 0.001$) than that observed in the normal population and considerably greater than any spontaneous activity observed in the dark (fig. 1). A striking feature was that in some patients, notably those operated upon many years previously, there was little or no spontaneous

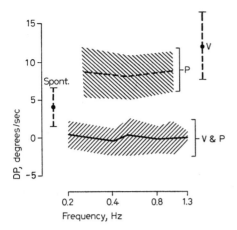

Fig. 1. Comparison of the directional preponderance (DP) of slow phase velocity in normals (n=12, —) and unilaterally labyrinthectomised (n=11, – – –) patients during voluntary (V) and passive (P) angular oscillation of the head about the longitudinal body axis. DP in patients has been normalized – left side lesion gave DP to left and vice versa. Limits indicate ± 1 SD.

nystagmus (<2°/sec), but still a significant directional preponderance (>8°/sec) could be observed in the oscillatory response. In the group of 4 patients who were tested pre-operatively there was no significant directional preponderance before labyrinthectomy offering no prior indication of vestibular dysfunction.

Experiment III

The same battery of experimental tests was also conducted on 2 patients with suspected bilateral canal paresis, a diagnosis which was indicated by a very low gain (<0.1) in the vestibulo-ocular response to passive whole-body oscillation and negligible response to caloric irrigation. However, in both patients the response to voluntary head movement showed a gain of 0.4–0.5. Following the evidence of *Dichgans et al.* [5] in monkeys, it was expected that these patients would exhibit a potentiated cervico-ocular response. The results, however, were equivocal in this respect, since in 1 patient there was no evidence of a significant response whereas in the other a compensatory reflex with a gain of approximately 0.3 was observed.

Saccadic Eye Movements

Experiments on normal subjects [1, 2] have indicated that stimulation of the vestibulo-ocular reflex alone is sufficient to elicit not only compensatory eye movements, but also saccades indistinguishable from those observed during visual target acquisition. The amplitude of the saccadic eye movement was found to be related to slow phase eye velocity.

In both groups of patients with vestibular dysfunction the amplitude of saccades was also related to slow phase eye velocity, even though the slow phase might be abnormal. Thus, in the immediate period following unilateral labyrinthectomy, when there was a marked spontaneous nystagmus, saccades were smaller and occurred later, or not at all, when the spontaneous activity interacted in an antagonistic manner with the slow phase eye velocity arising from the head-turning manoeuvre, and vice versa.

Visual Suppression of Inappropriate Eye Movement

The ability to suppress inappropriate reflex eye movements when fixating a head-fixed image during head movement was assessed in the 2 patients with bilateral canal paresis. Rather surprisingly, both patients experienced considerable difficulty as evidenced by the oculomotor response which contained both fast and slow phase activity. This is a clear indication of the consolidation of their adaptation to loss of labyrinthine function. The same patients, when fixating an earth-fixed object during head movement, produced effective compensatory slow phase eye movements up to a frequency of approximately 1.2 Hz, but thereafter the response broke down.

Conclusions

The results have demonstrated that when the response from one horizontal canal is completely absent there is a significant directional preponderance in the response to an oscillatory stimulus, even though there may be negligible spontaneous nystagmus because of the action of central adaptive mechanisms which counteract the unbalanced resting discharge emanating from the intact crista. Thus, any directional preponderance in the oculomotor response reflects an asymmetry in the response produced by the single remaining end organ which, in the normal subject, is balanced out by the effects of reciprocal innervation. The asymmetry could reflect a greater sensitivity of the end organ to excitatory as opposed to inhibitory stimuli (Ewald's 2nd law), a feature demonstrated by *Goldberg and Fernandez* [6] in the squirrel monkey.

Summary

Oculomotor response in the absence of vision was examined in 8 normal subjects, 11 unilaterally labyrinthectomised patients and 2 patients with suspected bilateral canal paresis. The experiments involved (a) voluntary oscillation of the head, (b) whole body oscillation on a turntable and (c) stimulation of neck afferents by oscillation of the body with the head fixed. In the patients with unilateral lesions there was a directional preponderance of the slow phase eye velocity towards the side of the lesion which differed significantly from that of the normal population. In the patients with bilateral paresis the oculomotor response to whole body oscillation was negligible, whereas the response to voluntary head movement had a mean gain of 0.45 and at high frequency could not be suppressed when viewing a head-fixed image. The saccadic activity during voluntary head movement was similar in all subjects and was correlated with slow phase velocity.

References

1   Barnes, G.R.: The role of the vestibular system in head-eye coordination. J. Physiol. *246:* 99–100P (1975).
2   Barnes, G.R.: The role of the vestibulo-ocular reflex in visual target acquisition. J. Physiol. *258:* 64–65P (1976).
3   Barnes, G.R. and Forbat, L.N.: Cervical and vestibular afferent control of oculomotor response in man (in press, 1978).
4   Benson, A.J.: Interaction between semicircular canals and gravireceptors; in Busby, Recent advances in aerospace medicine, pp. 249–261 (Reidel, Dordrecht 1970).
5   Dichgans, J.; Bizzi, E.; Morasso, P., and Tagliasco, V.: Mechanisms underlying recovery of eye-head coordination following bilateral labyrinthectomy in monkeys. Expl. Brain Res. *18:* 548–562 (1973).
6   Goldberg, J.M. and Fernandez, C.: Physiology of peripheral neurons innervating semicircular canals of the squirrel monkey. I. Resting discharge and response to constant acceleration. J. Neurophysiol. *39:* 635–648 (1971).

G.R. Barnes, PhD, RAF, Institute of Aviation Medicine, Farnborough, Hants (England)

Adv. Oto-Rhino-Laryng., vol. 25, pp. 202–207 (Karger, Basel 1979)

Optokinetic Nystagmus in Artificial Hemianopsy

T. Miyoshi, M. Shirato and S. Hiwatashi

Ear, Nose, and Throat Department, Fukui Red Cross Hospital, Fukui

Introduction

Fukuda and Tokita [3] stated that the retina of the rabbit showed unilaterality to optokinetic stimulus. It has, however, not yet been confirmed whether the human retina has unilaterality or not. *Barany* [2] described 2 cases of hemianopsy in which optokinetic nystagmus to the affected side was absent, in spite of the fact that the nystagmus to the healthy side was well induced. *Ishiguro* [5] concluded that, in hemianopsy, an affection of the optomotor tract disturbed the optokinetic nystagmus to the affected side, but a disorder of the optosensory tract had no influence upon the optokinetic nystagmus. But *Aso* [1] showed that covering half the visual field with a special glass disturbed the optokinetic nystagmus to the covered side. *Ohm* [8] examined 58 cases of hemianopsy and found that optokinetic nystagmus was well induced to both sides in 30 cases. In order to clarify these questions, artificial hemianopsy was produced by the visual-field-isolation method, which was reported at the last meeting.

Method

The equipment was the same as that described in the last report [7]. Half the visual field was blocked, in order to produce an artificial hemianopsy. The left eye of the test subject was covered with an eyepatch. Only the right eye was stimulated in both directions, to the right (nasotemporal) and to the left (temporonasal). The test subject placed his or her chin on the headrest to prevent head movement. The normal sight was also studied as a control. As it had already been stated that the foveal and peripheral retinas had quite different properties in relation to optokinetic stimulus, two sorts of hemianopsy, with or without foveal vision, were studied. The angles of view in each condition were restricted uniformly to 60° to equalize the stimuli. As a consequence, five visual conditions were tested – normal eye, nasal and temporal hemianopsy (foveal vision reserved) and nasal and temporal hemianopsy (foveal vision involved). To produce these test conditions, five black sheets (fig. 1) were used. A in figure 1 is the sheet for the normal eye with 60° of visual angle, B for nasal hemianopsy (foveal vision reserved), C for temporal hemianopsy (foveal vision reserved), D for nasal hemianopsy (foveal vision involved) and E for temporal hemianopsy (foveal vision involved) for the tested right eye. For the foveal vision, a visual angle of 20° for the central part was reserved or covered. Eye movement was picked up by $Zn-ZnSO_4$, bitemporal, skin electrodes. After DC amplification, the potential was divided between two circuits, one for recording on a polygraph and the other for driving the erasing device.

Eye movements and target traces were superimposed by the overlapping method described in the last report. Thanks to this overlapping method, the relationship between the moving target and the fixation point of vision in optokinetic nystagmus can be discussed. Three sorts of uniform velocities for optokinetic stimuli were used. They were 15, 30 and 60°/sec. 24 black stripes of 3° arranged at equal distances of 15° were projected on a white, semicylindrical screen in front of the test subjects.

Results

Five sorts of optokinetic stimuli were presented in random order. 5 normal persons, 4 males and 1 female, ranging in age from 26 to 50 years were tested. The typical results are demonstrated in figure 1. The velocity of stimulus in this figure is 30°/sec. When foveal vision is reserved, in cases of both temporal and nasal hemianopsy, optokinetic nystagmus is well induced, except with high-speed stimulation (60°/sec). The slow phases of optokinetic nystagmus coincide relatively well with the target trace. There is no difference between nystagmus induced by nasotemporal stimulation and that induced by temporonasal stimulation. There is also no distinct difference between nystagmus induced by foveopetal stimuli and that induced by foveofugal stimuli. There is no essential difference between nystagmus in the normal eye and that in hemianopsy in which foveal vision is reserved, except with high-speed stimulation. When the speed of stimulus is 60°/sec, the amplitude and slow-phase velocity are reduced, but the frequency is not so affected (fig. 2).

When the foveal vision is involved, on the contrary, there are remarkable differences in the resulting nystagmus. Nystagmus during foveofugal stimulation is quite different from that during other conditions. A remarkable change is seen in the nystagmus induced by foveofugal stimulation. The amplitude, slow-phase velocity and frequency of the nystagmus declined greatly even when the speed of stimulus is slow (fig. 2). Then nystagmus is very fine and irregular. The slow phase does not coincide

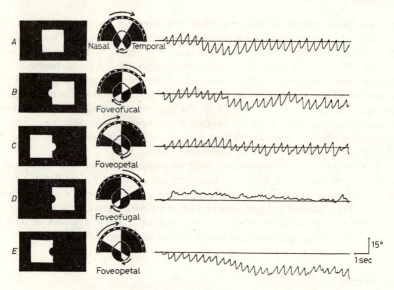

Fig. 1. Visual field and optokinetic nystagmus in artificial hemianopsy. *A* Normal eye. *B, C* Hemianopsy in which the foveal vision is reserved. *D, E* Hemianopsy in which foveal vision is involved. Nystagmus is suppressed in D (foveofugal stimulation).

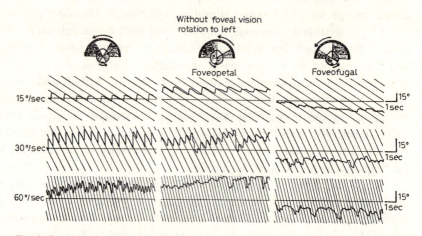

Fig. 2. Optokinetic nystagmus in hemianopsy in which the foveal vision is involved. Nystagmus is well induced by foveopetal stimulation but on the contrary, is fine and irregular with foveofugal stimulation. The eye velocity in the slow phase of hemianopsy is slower than that of the target, even at 15°/sec.

with the target movement and the beginning of the slow phase is very obtuse. During high-speed stimulation, the nystagmus vanishes and only target-seeking eye movements can be seen. During foveopetal stimulation, on the contrary, the nystagmus is not so affected (fig. 2). The slow-phase eye velocity in foveopetal cases is slower than that of the moving target, too. This velocity lag of the eye movement increases as the velocity of the target increases. However, the wave form is not so distorted. The returns of both components (slow and quick phases) are sharp enough. This fact indicates that the eye catches the next target exactly on the fovea.

There is no essential difference between optokinetic nystagmus induced by nasotemporal stimuli and that induced by temporonasal stimuli. There is also no noteworthy difference between the nystagmus in temporal hemianopsy and that in nasal hemianopsy.

Discussion

For the induction of optokinetic nystagmus, not only the fovea but also the peripheral retina is very important [4, 6, 7]. The retina of the rabbit reacts only to optokinetic stimulus in the nasopetal direction [3]. Investigation of optokinetic nystagmus in hemianopsy has revealed that nystagmus is well induced by stimulation to the affected side. However, no definite conclusion as to the reaction to stimulus to the healthy side has yet been established [2, 5, 8]. This confusion may arise from the lack of consideration of the conditions of foveal vision. Since the central and the peripheral retina are not the same histologically, because of distinct differences between the roles of foveal and peripheral vision [4] and of differences between the nystagmuses induced in foveal and peripheral vision [7], we have to consider whether the foveal vision is reserved or affected, in order to discuss the optokinetic nystagmus of hemianopsy.

In investigating the mechanism of optokinetic nystagmus, studies of hemianopsy are very worthwhile. Hitherto, the half-covered cylinder [5], half-masked glass or contact lenses have been used to produce hemianopsy artificially [1, 5]. These methods, however, are not accurate. They cannot produce a stable hemianopsy. In the discussion of the resulting nystagmus, the involvement of foveal vision has never been considered.

It is very clear from our results that consideration of foveal vision is very important in studies of optokinetic nystagmus in hemianopsy. A remarkable diminution of optokinetic nystagmus in hemianopsy can be seen only when the fovea is also involved and stimulated in the foveofugal direction. This result shows that the retina on the foveofugal side has only a small effect on the induced optokinetic nystagmus. There is no essential difference between optokinetic nystagmus in the normal eye and in hemianopsy in which the foveal vision is reserved. This fact also indicates that the retina on the foveofugal side has a weak effect upon induced optokinetic nystagmus. This fact is very advantageous for individuals. If the retina on the foveofugal side reacts powerfully, some targets on the foveofugal side will attract the eyes strongly to the rotating side, that is, in the opposite direction of the quick phase of optokinetic nystagmus. This must disturb the optokinetic nystagmus, which is an important physiological reaction. The slow-phase eye velocity of optokinetic nystagmus in the fovea involved in hemianopsy is slower than the velocity of the moving target, even when the eye is stimulated in the foveopetal direction. This fact indicates that foveal vision is indispensable for the production of the slow phase of optokinetic nystagmus.

Conclusion

The studies on optokinetic nystagmus in artificial hemianopsy reveal the following facts. (1) Temporal and nasal hemianopsy have the same properties in relation to optokinetic stimulus. (2) There is no essential difference between optokinetic nystagmus induced by nasotemporal and temporonasal stimulation. (3) When the foveal vision is reserved, there is no noteworthy difference between optokinetic nystagmus in hemianopsy induced by foveopetal and foveofugal stimulation. (4) In the case of hemianopsy in which the foveal vision is involved, nystagmus during foveofugal stimulation is very fine and irregular, in spite of the nystagmus being well induced during foveopetal stimulation. (5) The fovea is very important for the formation of the slow component of nystagmus. (6) Foveopetal movement of the image in the peripheral retina is very important for the formation of the quick component and is stronger than foveofugal movement in the peripheral retina as a stimulus to attract the eye.

Summary

Optokinetic nystagmus in cases of artificial hemianopsy was studied. Hemianopsy was produced by using a combination of a projector, an erasing device and DC ENG.

The effect of the condition of foveal vision in hemianopsy, whether reserved or involved, was discussed. When foveal vision was reserved, nystagmus during stimulation in cases of hemianopsy was essentially the same as in the normal eye. In cases of hemianopsy in which foveal vision was involved, there was a remarkable difference between the nystagmus induced by foveofugal stimulation and that induced by foveopetal stimulation. In the former case the nystagmus was very fine and irregular, in spite of the fact that the nystagmus was well induced (it was nearly the same as in the normal eye in the latter case). Foveal vision is very important for the formation of the slow component of optokinetic nystagmus. Foveopetal movement of the image on the peripheral retina is very important for the formation of the quick component. Foveofugal movement on the peripheral retina has, on the contrary, only a small effect in attracting the eye.

References

1   Aso, T.: Analytic observation on the labyrinthine nystagmus by electronystagmography. Acta med. biol. 2: 93–112 (1956).

2   Barany, R.: Zur Klinik und Theorie des Eisenbahnnystagmus. Acta oto-lar. 3: 260–265 (1921).

3   Fukuda, T. und Tokita, T.: Über die Beziehung der Richtung der optokinetischen Reize zu den Reflextypen der Augen und Skelettmuskeln. Acta oto-lar. 48: 415–424 (1957).

4   Hood, J.D.: Observations upon the neurological mechanisms of optokinetic nystagmus with especial reference to the contribution of peripheral vision. Acta oto-lar. 63: 208–215 (1967).

5   Ishiguro, E.: Some observations on the optokinetic nystagmus. (In Japanese) Niigata med. J. 73: 1664–1683 (1959).

6   Miyoshi, T. and Pfaltz, C.R.: Studies on the correlation between optokinetic stimulation and induced nystagmus. 2. The influence of the visual fields upon the optokinetic response. ORL 35: 350–362 (1973).

7   Miyoshi, T.; Shirato, M., and Hiwatashi, S.: Foveal and peripheral vision in optokinetic nystagmus; in Hood, Vestibular mechanisms in health and disease, pp. 294–301 (Academic Press, London 1978).

8   Ohm, J.: Über den Einfluss der gleichseitigen Halbblindheit auf den optokinetischen Nystagmus. Arch. Ophthal., Berlin 135: 200–219 (1936).

T. Miyoshi, MD, Kyoto University, Faculty of Medicine,
Department of Otolaryngology, Sakyo-ku, Kyoto 606 (Japan)

Adv. Oto-Rhino-Laryng., vol. 25, pp. 208–213 (Karger, Basel 1979)

The Mechanism of Inhibition of Caloric Nystagmus by Eye Closure

S. Takemori, H. Moriyama and G. Totsuka

Department of Neurotology, Toranomon Hospital, Tokyo

Introduction

It is well known that vestibular nystagmus is inhibited by eye closure [1, 3]. Eye position [1] or alertness [2] during eye closure influences the vestibular nystagmus.

The purpose of this paper is to clarify the mechanism of nystagmus inhibition by eye closure.

Methods

24 normal adults and 324 clinical cases were tested. DC recordings of monocular, horizontal and vertical, eye movements were made by using electronystagmography (ENG). Horizontal eye velocity was also recorded. The electroencephalogram was recorded stimultaneously with the eye movements, in order to measure the α-wave responses of the occipital areas during eye closure.

Caloric nystagmus was evoked by injection 20 ml of ice water into the external auditory canal and recorded by ENG with the eyes covered in darkness. The effect of eye closure on caloric nystagmus was tested and recorded while the caloric nystagmus was provoked.

Results

Normal Eye Movements during Eye Closure. When the eyes were closed, they were suddenly adducted $13 \pm 5°$ and elevated $55 \pm 11°$. These movements associated with eye closure were normal responses.

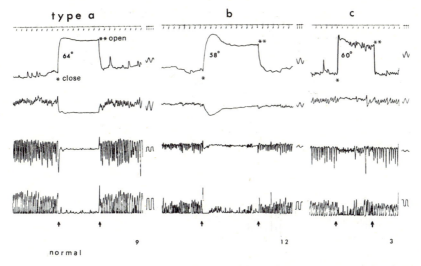

Fig. 1. Three types of eye movements associated with eye closure during caloric nystagmus in normal adults. The top row of traces shows the time marks (1 mark/sec), the second row of traces presents the DC recordings of vertical eye movements (right eye), the third row of traces shows the DC recordings of horizontal eye movements (right eye) and the fourth row of traces presents the horizontal eye velocity. The bottom traces represent the horizontal slow-phase velocity of caloric nystagmus. Calibrations are shown on the right, 10° for eye movements, 20°/sec for eye velocity. These are the same in figures 1, 2 and 3.

There were four types of vertical eye-movement responses during eye closure: (a) holding the eye position up, (b) fluctuating movements around an elevated eye position, (c) gradual downward turning, (d) sudden downward turning. Type a was seen in 9 people (37.5%); type b was seen in 12 people (59%); type c was seen in 3 people (12.5%) (fig. 1). However, the type d was not seen in normal adults.

Effect of Eye Position on Nystagmus. Nystagmus was inhibited when the eyes were turned in the slow-phase direction and enhanced when the eyes were turned in the direction of the quick phase. Horizontal nystagmus was suppressed when the eyes were elevated. This suppression depended on the degree of eyeball elevation. The suppression was present both in involuntary eye elevation during eye closure and in voluntary eye deviation with the eyes open in darkness (fig. 2). This suppression from the vertical eye position was abolished when the eyes returned to their initial position.

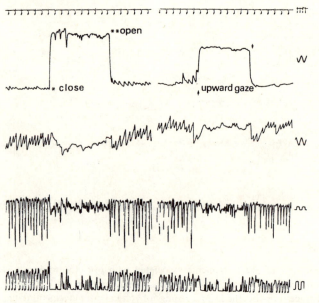

Fig. 2. Suppression of caloric nystagmus by eye closure and upward gaze.

Effect of Eye Closure on Caloric Nystagmus. Adductive and upward eye deviation were seen with the eyes closed. These movements were also observed when the eyes were closed during caloric nystagmus. The resulting eye elevation greatly inhibited caloric nystagmus; the horizontal eye position affected it less. This inhibition was visible in measurements of slow- and quick-phase velocities, frequency and amplitude.

The strength of the eye closure affected the vertical deviation of the eyes and stronger eye closure caused less fluctuation. However, the type of vertical eye movement was unchanged by stronger eye closure (fig. 3).

Effect of Eye Position on Caloric Nystagmus during Eye Closure. When the eyes turned to the right or left during eye closure, the vertical eye position fluctuated. When the subjects were required to move their eyes upward or downward during eye closure, the vertical eye position also fluctuated. However, the type of vertical eye position caused by eye closure was unchanged by the eye position during closure. That is, the eye positions during closure influenced the vertical eye position. However, they could not change

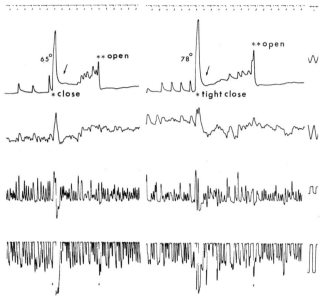

Fig. 3. Effect of closing the eyes on caloric nystagmus. Larger, vertical eye deviations were caused by stronger eye closure. However, the type of vertical eye movements caused by stronger eye closure was the same as that caused by light eye closure.

the type of vertical eye position caused by closure. Therefore, when the vertical eye position fluctuates during closure, stronger eye closure should be required to confirm the responses.

Duration of Eye Closure. For people showing type c or d responses, the onset of turning down was 1–5 sec after eye closure. Therefore, eye closure for 5–10 sec was enough to observe this phenomenon.

Reproducibility of Upward Eye Deviation Caused by Eye Closure. The subjects were required to close their eyes 5–10 times. The type of vertical eye movement responses associated with eye closure was the same in each trial.

Caloric Nystagmus and Mental Calculation during Eye Closure. Caloric nystagmus was enhanced by mental calculation. During mental calculation with the eyes closed, most subjects turned their eyes downward toward their initial position. In other subjects who maintained their upward eye position during mental calculation, their caloric nystagmus was greatly inhibited.

α-Activity and Caloric Nystagmus during Eye Closure. α-Activity was evoked by eye closure and by eye elevation. α-Waves were also seen during mental calculation with the eyes closed, with or without maintained, upward, eye elevation. However, α-activity was not observed with the eyes open. There was no apparent correlation between α-activity and nystagmus inhibition associated with eye closure.

Effects of Eyelid on Caloric Nystagmus. Three cases of Bell's facial palsy were tested. Caloric nystagmus showed the same inhibition during closure of the eyelid on the normal side as was shown on the affected side, where the eyelid remained open.

Discussion

There are many reports of the effect of eye closure on caloric nystagmus or rotatory nystagmus. *Ohm* [3], *Mahoney et al.* [1] and *Naito et al.* [2] reported that vestibular nystagmus was inhibited by eye closure. However, the mechanism of inhibition of vestibular nystagmus by eye closure has remained obscure.

Tjernström [5] reported that the vertical eye position during eye closure greatly inhibited caloric nystagmus. We observed such an effect in the present study. When the eyes were held in their initial, upward, eye position during eye closure (type a), caloric nystagmus was greatly inhibited throughout the eye closure period. When there was downward turning (type c), the caloric-nystagmus inhibition was released. Horizontal eye position affected caloric nystagmus to a lesser extent during eye closure.

When caloric nystagmus was enhanced during mental calculation, the eyes turned downward. α-Activity was recorded during eye closure whether the caloric nystagmus was inhibited or not.

Thus, caloric nystagmus is greatly influenced by upward eye deviation during eye closure. Upward eye deviation is controlled by the oculomotor nucleus, which is connected with the cerebellum, medial longitudinal fasciculus, inner ear, vestibular nuclei and also the cerebrum. Abnormal downward turning of the eyes has been observed in cases of cerebellar or inner ear lesions [4]. The mechanism of nystagmus suppression by eye closure seems to result mainly from an interaction of these structures.

Therefore, the condition with eyes closed is different from that with eyes covered. The purpose of covering the eyes is to eliminate visual fixation. If the eye position caused by closure returns to the initial position, its condition is the same as that with eyes covered.

Summary

24 normal adults and 324 clinical cases were examined, for the purpose of shedding light on the mechanism of inhibition of caloric nystagmus by eye closure.

When the eyes were closed, an eye was suddenly adducted $13 \pm 5°$ and elevated $55 \pm 11°$. These adductive and upward eye movements were normal responses caused by eye closure.

Caloric nystagmus was inhibited by upward eye deviation. With the turning down of the vertical eye position, the caloric-nystagmus inhibition was released.

During eye closure, there were four types of vertical eye-movement responses: (a) holding the eye position up, (b) fluctuation around an upward eye position, (c) gradual downward turning, (d) sudden downward turning. Types a, b and c were seen in normal subjects. However, type d was not seen in normal people.

References

1   Mahoney, J.L.; Harlan, W.L., and Bickford, R.G.: Visual and other factors in-
    fluencing caloric nystagmus in normal subjects. Archs Otolar. *66:* 46–53 (1957).
2   Naito, T.; Tatsumi, T., et al.: The effect of eye closure upon nystagmus. Acta oto-
    lar. *179:* suppl., pp. 72–85 (1963).
3   Ohm, J.: Über den Einfluss des Sehens auf den vestibulären Drehnystagmus und
    Nachnystagmus. Z. Hals- Nasen- Ohrenheilk. *16:* 521–540 (1926).
4   Takemori, S.; Ono, M., and Maeda, T.: Eye closure and caloric nystagmus inhibition
    (in press, 1978).
5   Tjernström, Ö.: Nystagmus inhibition as an effect of eye closure. Acta oto-lar. *75:*
    408–418 (1973).

S. Takemori, MD, Department of Neurotology, Toranomon Hospital,
Toranomon 2-2-2, Minatu-ku, Tokyo 107 (Japan)

Adv. Oto-Rhino-Laryng., vol. 25, pp. 214–220 (Karger, Basel 1979)

The Tonic Oculomotor Function of the Cervical Joint and Muscle Receptors

George Botros

Ear, Nose and Throat Department, Ain Shams University, Cairo

Introduction

Cervical afferents have been shown to excite oculomotor and vestibular neurons. Thus, depolarizing potential has been induced in abducent motor neurons by ipsilateral dorsal-root stimulation, which activated the contralateral vestibular neurons intercalated with the vestibular abducens reflex pathway [4]. The neurons in the left internal rectus muscle display a more tonic discharge pattern when the head deviation is to the left [8]. Stimulation of neck muscles by weak electronic stimuli in the rabbit increases the frequency of the OKN [5]. The cervical joint receptors responsible for neck-induced oculomotor activity are located in the upper neck joints, especially at the atlanto-axial and atlanto-occipital [6]. The afferent information enters the spinal cord via dorsal roots C1 to C3 and possibly C4. Both the spray type of receptors found in the connective tissue of the capsules and the Golgi type found in the ligaments are slowly adaptive. The muscles which rotate the HC to one side lie on both sides of the neck, the obliquus capitus inferior, the rectus capitus posterior major and the splenius capitus of one side acting with the sternomastoid of the other side. The muscle receptors which excite the vestibular and reticular units bilaterally are the Golgi tendon organs and secondary spindles and not the la pathway [7]. Cases of peripheral labyrinthine lesions with no evidence of CNS and cervical abnormality have been examined with a view to elucidating the functional implications.

Material and Methods

The stimulus to joint receptors is the stretching of the joint ligaments and capsules in the head-chin position 45° to the left (HCL) and to the right (HCR). With the subject

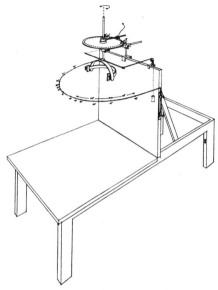

Fig. 1. The head-holder.

seated, his head was adjusted in a special head-holder (fig. 1) fixed to the head of the table. The position of the HC in degrees was given by an electric contact, providing a visible indication to the observer, a half circle of wire adjustable to eye level and 1 m in diameter, with its center at the bridge of the nose, was marked in degrees for gaze deviation. Gaze deviation was recorded with the head in three positions (head-chin center (HCC), left (HCL) and right (HCR) and with three directions of gaze in each position (eyes looking straight ahead, eyes deviating 30° to the right and eyes deviating 30° to the left). Gaze deviation was measured in light and darkness for 10 sec and with the eyes closed.

OKAN. A large drum 1.5 m in diameter, with black stripes 2 cm wide at intervals of 10°, could be rotated at 90°/sec⁻¹. Recording was carried out in the three positions of the HC with eyes looking straight ahead.

To induce isometric contraction of the neck muscles, a transverse rod was fixed to the vertical axis of the holder. To the end of the rod on either side, a 1-kg weight was attached by a cord directed backwards round a V pulley fixed to the top of the table. With the weight on either side, the subject was asked to counteract the force by contracting the muscles which rotate the HC to the opposite side and keep his HC in the center position, as indicated by the electric contact. Gaze fixation was recorded in HCC in the three directions of gaze with (1) the muscles which rotate the HC to the right (MR) and (2) the muscles which rotate the HC to the left (ML).

Recording in HCC with MR and ML was also carried out, using a small OKN drum 15 cm in diameter with black stripes 2 cm wide at intervals of 8°. Speeds of 20 and 40°/sec were used. Caloric tests were performed according to the sequence of Fitzgerald and Hallpike. The irrigation was for 30 sec. The tests were carried out in darkness with

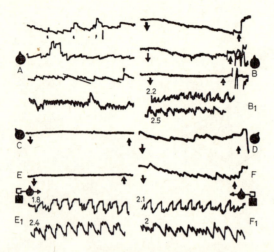

Fig. 2. Case 1. Electro-oculograms of gaze fixation in this and the following cases were made at 10-sec intervals in darkness (marked in the traces by downward arrow for light off and upward arrow for light on). (A) HCC. Caloric test. Paralysis of left canal and left utricle. Note right nystagmus in L.44. (B) HCC. Gaze fixation demonstrated labyrinthine, oculomotor asymmetry by 2nd degree nystagmus to right in top and middle traces; lower trace shows maintained left gaze. (B1) OKN frequency; left 2.2, right 2.5. Oculomotor changes induced by head position. (C) HCL towards left paralyzed canal. No change in left gaze. (D) HCR towards right-active canal; enhancement of 1st degree nystagmus to right. Oculomotor changes induced by muscle contraction. (E) MR in line with paralyzed, left utricle; no change in left gaze. (E1) Left OKN is distorted, frequency 1.8. Right OKN curtailment of slow-phase frequency 2.4. (F) ML in line with active, right utricle; enhancement of 1st degree, right nystagmus. (F1) Enhancement of the slow phase of the right OKN with diminution of frequency to 2/sec. Frequency of left OKN 2.1.

open eyes, the subject fixating his finger at the center of the circular ring of wire. Electro-oculography was used to record eye movements. The electrodes were chloridized silver discs 5 mm in diameter. They were placed at the outer canthi of the eyes. The subject was grounded by a third electrode fixed to the forehead. The Elema MT 12 was used for DC amplification. The recorder was the Elema Minograph 24. On the tracing, upward deviations from the baseline registered eye movements to the right and downward deviation eye movements to the left.

Results and Discussion

Oculomotor Changes Induced in Different Head Positions

The HC to one side induced compensatory tone (ipsilateral nystagmus), which depended on the function of the horizontal canal of that side. In

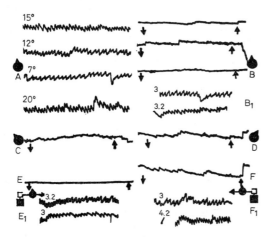

Fig. 3. Case 2. (A) HCC. Caloric test. Left canal and left, utricular paresis. (B) HCC. Gaze fixation demonstrated labyrinthine, oculomotor asymmetry by 2nd degree nystagmus to right in upper and middle traces. Lower trace shows maintained left gaze. (B1) OKN frequency: left 3.2 right 3/sec. Oculomotor changes induced by head positions. (C) HCL towards paretic, left canal. Left gaze shows fine, 1st degree nystagmus to left. (D) HCR towards active, right canal; enhancement of 1st degree nystagmus to right. Oculomotor changes induced by muscle contraction. (E) MR in line with paretic, left utricle; no change in left gaze. (E1) OKN frequency: left 3.2, right 3. (F) ML in line with active, right utricle, enhancement of 1st degree, right nystagmus. (F1) Frequency of right OKN was increased by 1 beat/sec to 4.2. Frequency of left OKN 3.

cases 1 and 2, with a functioning, right, horizontal canal, HCR induced compensatory tone to the left, which enhanced the existing, spontaneous, right-beating nystagmus. In case 1 (fig. 2), with paralysis of the left canal, there was no compensatory tone to the right (hence no nystagmus to the left) in HCL. In case 2 (fig. 3), with a paretic left canal, first-degree nystagmus to the left was induced in HCL. In case 3 (fig. 4), there were weak caloric responses and a predominance of the right labyrinth. HCR toward the supposed, active, right canal did not induce nystagmus to the right. HCL towards the supposed, weak canal induced a first-degree nystagmus to the left. According to *Dichgans* [2], neck afferences may become significant during the process of recovery from vestibular lesions. Combined stimulation with whole-field visual stimuli (large drum) showed the compensatory tone in both directions. The duration of the right and left OKAN was much increased in the HCR and HCL positions respectively. Circular vection was also induced; it was not present in HCC. This demonstrates the integration

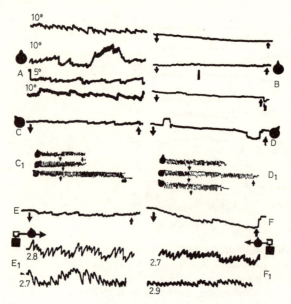

Fig. 4. Case 3. (A) HCC. Caloric test. Weak response with predominance of right labyrinth. (B) HCC. Gaze fixation showed no labyrinthine, oculomotor asymmetry. Fixation is maintained in the three directions of gaze. Oculomotor changes induced by head positions. (C) HCL. towards supposed, weak, left canal. 1st degree nystagmus to left. (C1) Left OKAN, starting at downward arrows. Top trace shows the duration in HCC. Bottom trace shows the increase of the duration in HCL. (D) HCR towards supposed, active, right canal; right gaze shows no definite response. (D1) Right OKAN starting at downward arrows. Top trace shows the duration in HCC. Middle trace shows the increase of the duration in HCR. Oculomotor changes induced by muscle contraction. (E) MR in line with left utricle. 1st degree nystagmus to left. (E1) OKN frequency: left 2.7, right 2.8/sec. (F) ML in line with right utricle. Tonic deviation to left with 1st degree nystagmus to right. (F1) OKN frequency: left 2.7, right 2.9.

of the cervical joint afferents with the vestibular and whole-retina visual pathway in the perception of self-rotation [1]. Type-1 vestibular neurons in the medial vestibular nucleus are distinctly facilitated by single shocks to the contralateral neck joints [4]. Type-1 neurons which were excited by ipsilateral acceleration were excited by whole-field stripes moving contra-laterally [3].

The oculomotor change induced by isometric contraction of the cervical muscles which rotate the HC to one side induces ipsilateral oculomotor tone (contralateral nystagmus), which depends on the function of the utricle acting in the same direction. In cases 1 and 2, with a functioning right utricle, the contraction of the muscles which rotate the HC to the left induced ipsilateral tone to the left, which enhanced the existing nystagmus to the right. The muscle-induced tone to the left in case 2 increased the frequency of the right OKN by 1 beat/sec. In case 1, it enhanced some of the pursuit phases to the left at the expense of the frequency, which was diminished by 0.5/sec. In case 1, with paralysis of the left utricle, there was no muscle-induced tone to the right. The left OKN showed distortion of the slow phases to the right with diminution of the frequency. There was curtailment of the slow pursuit phases to the left of OKN to the right. In this case, the inference is that there was excitation of the tonic, reticular units in the absence of the vestibular component.

In case 2, with a paretic left utricle, although there was no muscle-induced tone to the right, there was no distortion of the OKN to the left. In case 3, the cumulative amplitude of the muscle-induced tone to the left is larger than that to the right, demonstrating the predominance of the right utricle. There was no change in the frequency of the OKN. The changes in OKN demonstrate that muscle afferents are integrated with the vestibular and central, retinal, visual pathways in the pursuit tracking system. The tonic neck reflexes interact with the otolith inputs at the level of the brain stem [2].

The oculomotor responses of the central vestibular organization to stimulation of cervical joint and muscle receptors evaluate the ampullopetal function of the horizontal canal and utricle of the same side respectively and separately. Both functions are evaluated conjointly with hot caloric stimulation of the peripheral labyrinth. This also shows that the activity of the central vestibular neurons depends upon the tonic, afferent activity of the peripheral labyrinth.

Summary

Cases of peripheral labyrinthine lesions were examined by stimulation of the cervical joint and muscle receptors. Head-chin (HC) position to one side induced compensatory oculomotor tone (ipsilateral nystagmus), which depended on the function of the horizontal canal of that side. This compensatory tone increased the duration of the optokinetic afternystagmus (OKAN), with stripes moving contralaterally to the HC position. Isometric contraction of the muscles which rotate the HC to one side induced ipsilateral oculomotor tone (contralateral nystagmus), which depended on the function of the utricle acting in the same direction. In one case, the muscle-induced tone increased the frequency of the OKN with the slow phase in the same direction; in another, it prolonged the slow-phase pursuit interval. In the absence of a vestibular component, distortion of the OKN was induced.

References

1 Dichgans, J. and Brandt, T.: The psychophysics of visually induced perception of self motion and tilt; in Schmitt and Worden, Neurosciences: third study program, pp. 123–129 (Massachusetts Institute of Technology Press, Cambridge 1974).

2 Dichgans, J.: Spinal afferences to the oculomotor system. Physiological and clinical aspects; in Lennerstrand and Bachy-Rita, Basic mechanism of ocular motility and their clinical application, pp. 299–302 (Pergamon Press, Oxford 1975).

3 Henn, V.S.; Young, I.R., and Finleye, C.: Vestibular nucleus units in alert monkeys are also influenced by moving visual scenes. Brain Res. 71: 144–149 (1974).

4 Hikosaka, O. and Maeda, M.: Cervical effects on abducens motor neurons and the interaction with vestibulo-ocular reflex. Expl. Brain Res. 18: 512–530 (1973).

5 Hinoki, M.; Hini, J.; Okada, S.; Ishida, Y.; Koike, S., and Schizuku, S.: Optic organ and cervical proprioceptors in maintenance of body equilibrium. Acta oto-lar. suppl. 330, pp. 169–184 (1975).

6 McCough, G.P.; Deering, I.D., and Ling, T.H.: Location of receptors for tonic neck reflexes. J. Neurophysiol. 14: 191 (1951).

7 Pompeiano, O.: Spino-vestibular relations. Anatomical and physiological aspects. Prog. Brain Res. 37: 280 (1972).

8 Schaefer, K.P.; Meyer, D.L.; Buttner, U., and Schott, D.: Effect of head position on oculomotor discharge patterns in rabbits; in Lennerstrand and Bachy-Rita, Basic mechanisms of ocular motility and their clinical application, pp. 457–459 (Pergamon Press, Oxford 1975).

G. Botros, MD, 80, Gamhoria Street, Cairo (Egypt)

Closing Remarks

In my capacity as a former president of this society, and as a professor emeritus of this university, I have the honour and privilege of closing this symposium with a few words.

This international symposium is devoted to the memory of Robert Bárány, distinguished pioneer in the field of vestibular research, and first professor of otorhinolaryngology at the University of Uppsala. But let us not forget our president; *Hans Engström* arranged a Bárány symposium here in Uppsala for the last time. Professor *Engström* retires at the end of this year.

As you are all aware, the Bárány medal is awarded by the Faculty of Medicine once every five years. Thus the attention of vestibular researchers the world over is focused on Uppsala University every fifth year.

Our Society was founded to increase international cooperation in our field, to stimulate otoneurological research, and to arrange vestibular symposiums.

Last year, our University celebrated its 500th anniversary, and on that occasion established extensive international scientific contacts. We are honoured that this respected institution and many other enterprises have chosen to sponsor our symposium. Uppsala is the city in which scientific pioneers – such as Olof Rudbeck and Carl Linnaeus – lived and worked. A city steeped in an atmosphere of history and tradition. A city pervaded by centuries of civilisation.

On behalf of all the participants I would like to thank the organizers for this agreeable meeting and excellent arrangements. We are honoured and privileged this day to pay special tribute to *Hans Engström* – a man whose entire life has been devoted to scientific research, the fruits of which are known throughout the world. A man who has made great sacrifices to enable this Society to grow and develop. We wish him more many successful years of scientific work into the symbol of the century – space research.

We also wish to thank our general secretary, *Jan Stahle,* for his tireless efforts. *Jan* has gained an international reputation as an excellent organizer and first-rate scientist. We are happy to see him as our new president, successfully leading the Bárány Society for many years to come.

I cannot conclude without expressing our gratitude to the other members of the organizing committee who invested untold effort in ensuring that this symposium was stimulating and beneficial to all of us. I am certain that the memory of this occasion will remain with us for some time.

Arne Sjöberg, MD
Stockholm

Subject Index